Praise for *Rhythm and Touch*

"I first discovered Anthony Arnold's *Rhythm and Touch* nearly a dec... .go, when searching for just the right textbook to accompany the Introduction to Craniosacral Therapy classes I taught at the Center for Natural Wellness School of Massage Therapy in Albany, New York. Even in the book's original small format, Arnold presented, through text, illustrations, and photos, the perfect blend of what it takes to be a successful craniosacral therapist: compassion; presence; knowledge of oneself and the human body; the ability to slow down and listen; and, of course, curiosity and enthusiasm.

"This new edition of the book offers even more. With his usual clarity, Arnold has expanded on the fundamentals of craniosacral therapy, and even pushed ahead into more advanced material, including specific techniques for the face and jaw. Equally valuable are his inclusion of case studies, discussion of therapeutic dialoguing, and his graceful, practical suggestions for both teaching and learning. Throughout, Arnold reminds us that what is paramount to any healing practice is the intentional well-being of the practitioner. For new and emerging craniosacral practitioners, Anthony Arnold's *Rhythm and Touch* continues to be the ideal textbook."

— Margery Chessare, LMT, BCST, craniosacral therapist and educator, founder and codirector, Saratoga Integrative Practitioners Network

"*Rhythm and Touch* is the best basic book on craniosacral therapy that I know of. We have been using this wonderful book since the start of our school almost twelve years ago. It is indispensable. We have not used any other book, although we have looked at several. Craniosacral Therapy is not an easy course but this book makes it understandable for the students."

— Craig S. Anderson, LMT, director, Ogden Institute of Massage Therapy

"This is the best book we've ever used for our craniosacral training. It is comprehensive and easy to follow. Our students and instuctors have only good things to say about it. Thank you for making this book available to our school."

— Dr. Jack Weaver, director, Northwest Academy of Healing Arts

Rhythm
and Touch

THE FUNDAMENTALS OF CRANIOSACRAL THERAPY

Anthony P. Arnold, PhD

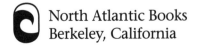
North Atlantic Books
Berkeley, California

Published by
North Atlantic Books
P.O. Box 12327
Berkeley, California 94712

Cover foreground image ©iStockphoto.com/Yanik Chauvin
Cover background image ©iStockphoto.com/Randy Plett
Cover and book design by Jan Camp
Interior drawings by Pamela Balanag and Anthony P. Arnold
Interior photographs by Pamela Balanag, Asti Hagenbach,
    and Gayan Sylvie Winter
Author photograph by Gayan Sylvie Winter
Printed in the United States of America

Rhythm and Touch: The Fundamentals of Craniosacral Therapy is sponsored by the Society for the Study of Native Arts and Sciences, a nonprofit educational corporation whose goals are to develop an educational and cross-cultural perspective linking various scientific, social, and artistic fields; to nurture a holistic view of arts, sciences, humanities, and healing; and to publish and distribute literature on the relationship of mind, body, and nature.

North Atlantic Books' publications are available through most bookstores. For further information, visit our Web site at www.northatlanticbooks.com or call 800-733-3000.

Library of Congress Cataloging-in-Publication Data

Arnold, Anthony P., 1938-
  Rhythm and touch : the fundamentals of craniosacral therapy / Anthony Arnold.
     p. ; cm.
  Presents material from: Rhythm & touch / Anthony P. Arnold. c1995.
  ISBN 978-1-55643-819-6
  1. Craniosacral therapy. I. Arnold, Anthony P., 1938- Rhythm & touch. II. Title.
  [DNLM: 1. Manipulation, Osteopathic—methods. 2. Sacrum. 3. Skull. WB 940 A752r 2009]
  RZ399.C73A76 2009
  615.8′2—dc22
                                                                    2008053431

1 2 3 4 5 6 7 8 9 UNITED 14 13 12 11 10 09

To my wife, Gayan Sylvie Winter

Acknowledgments

My first craniosacral course was a revelation, thanks to Bhadrena Tschumi. Other teachers and mentors joined her, inspiring and guiding me in my first years exploring craniosacral therapy. Charles Gilliam, Dick MacDonald, and Judith Sullivan stand out. Colleagues and friends at the Upledger Brain and Spinal Cord Dysfunction Center and in our advanced training helped me along the way as I made the move from psychotherapy to body-oriented therapy.

Teaching craniosacral has been one of the greatest learning experiences of my life. Thanks to Daniel Agustoni for the beginning years at Sphinx Workshops in Basel, Switzerland. Blessings and many thanks to Karin Duttke, Ursula Spescha, Burkhard Behm, Elfi Schaller, Theresa Dätwyler, and Gudrun Schmidt for the years of support, collaboration, and friendship as we learned more fully what we were doing as therapists, teachers, and students.

I wrote the original edition of this book on the urging of my wife, Gayan, and her agent and collaborator, Wulfing von Rohr. Thanks to them and to Goldmann/Bertelsmann Publishing for that beginning. The interest of a few schools and teachers has kept the manuscript edition alive in English.

After years of learning from clients, students, and colleagues, I am able to review and add to the previous editions. Deepest thanks to the people at North Atlantic Books for bringing a new life to this book.

CONTENTS

ILLUSTRATIONS

Part I

Part II

PREFACE

In the early nineties, I wrote *Rhythm and Touch* as an introductory guide to craniosacral therapy. My goal was to present in clear language the fundamentals of a profound and effective approach to human healing. First published in German translation, it was soon available in English and Italian. That original text was well received by students, teachers, and experienced practitioners. In down-to-earth language, it offers a cohesive, systematic guide to the fundamentals of craniosacral therapy.

Over the next few years, I developed a second text, presenting the material for a second course. Eventually, both works were combined in a single volume. Though this was published in German translation in 2001, it has been available only as a manuscript copy in English.

The following two parts present materials for a first and a second course of craniosacral therapy. In each part, the attitude, sensitivity, and responsiveness of the therapist is presented as a continuously important aspect of the healing interaction.

Part 1 constitutes the groundwork. Extensive descriptions and exercises describe an approach to the whole body and head. This gives a comprehensive basis for a beginning practice. The full treatment protocol can be very helpful in the relief of chronic pain and restricted motion. Moreover, these steps constitute a framework for learning. Through repetition, the beginning practitioner develops sensitivity of touch and an ever-growing appreciation of the power of the soft, respectful contact embodied in craniosacral therapy. A helpful summary of the treatment protocol is included in appendix 1.

Part 2 presumes the groundwork of the first section, as well as some months of experience, which deepens and softens the touch. Part 2 delves deeper into the relationship of the bones of the cranial base. It presents detailed information on possible constrictions and traditional approaches to release in this region.

In addition, part 2 describes the interaction of the bones of the mouth and face. These are important extensions forward from the cranial vault. Release in this area often eases stiffness and discomfort that may accumulate as we confront daily life.

Equally important, the second part encourages a deeper appreciation of the quality of touch, and a more profound respect for and trust in the healing capability of the individual.

INTRODUCTION

Near the beginning of the twentieth century, a young osteopathic physician in the midwestern United States, William G. Sutherland, became fascinated by the structure and function of the bones of the skull. In particular, he wondered about the usefulness of the sutures, or seams, between the bones. Despite a British and American tradition viewing the bones as a rigid structure, he postulated that the soft connective tissue at the suture must allow movement and adjustment among the cranial bones.

Initially he experimented on himself, constructing a device to apply pressure against specific locations on his skull. He carefully recorded his observations of the physical symptoms he experienced. Meanwhile, his wife kept a journal of the psychological impact of his experiments.

At times, his reactions were quite distressing, and took further time for recovery. However, Sutherland established that the skull is flexible enough to admit clear responses to various external pressures.

As he proceeded, Dr. Sutherland discovered that he could feel, or palpate, a subtle rhythmic movement among the cranial bones, and along the spine to its end at the sacrum. This movement occurred independently of the motions produced by the heart and lungs.

Working with himself and his medical patients, Sutherland discovered uniform patterns of rhythm, as well as specific deviations from the normal rhythm. He learned that he could assist in easing these deviations by applying external pressures in association with the natural movements of the cranial bones.

Thus, he founded Cranial Osteopathy, a therapeutic tradition that has persisted to this day. Yet, the therapeutic application of his work was accepted by only a few of his fellow osteopathic physicians. In general,

American medical and anatomical teaching continued to maintain that the sutures between the cranial bones become calcified and rigid during normal development. And the patience required to perceive the subtle cranial movement appears to have been more than could be expended by busy medical students and researchers. For much of the twentieth century, little was done to pursue Sutherland's research, and relatively few people benefited from his discoveries. In fact, there has been a great move away from hands-on contact between doctor and patient. Modern medical practice relies increasingly on technical instrumentation and expensive medications.

Upledger

In the 1970s, another osteopathic physician, John E. Upledger, found his interest in cranial rhythm suddenly aroused. Osteopathic medicine in America teaches, along with a full medical curriculum, an array of manipulative techniques for correcting somatic abnormalities that may underlie or enhance a disease process. As a student at the same school attended by Dr. Sutherland, Dr. Upledger and his classmates were taught cranial manipulative techniques. Nevertheless, most dismissed them as of little importance.

Many years later, as a practicing physician in Florida, Dr. Upledger was assisting a neurologist in an operation on one of his patients. He reports being astounded to note an unexpected movement in the tissue protecting the spinal cord. This experience led to a renewed study of cranial osteopathy. With new interest, he pursued the work of Sutherland and those who followed him at the Cranial Academy.

An appointment to the faculty at Michigan State University provided additional stimulus. Dr. Upledger benefited from the interest, the questions, and even the skepticism of his colleagues. An Israeli biophysicist set out to puncture Dr. Upledger's notion of an energy exchange between client and therapist. The biophysicist's careful work revealed that clear and eventually predictable electrical currents were associated with evaluation, treatment, and resolution of physiological symptoms. His measurements and continual questioning helped Dr. Upledger to clarify and express consciously his intuitive treatment procedures.

When Dr. Upledger began to work with autistic children in an institution, he enlisted students and laypeople to assist him. He shared basic craniosacral practices, benefited from the observations of his assistants, and experimented with many hands assisting in a single treatment. Until then, cranial work had been considered the bastion of the medical profession. However, Dr. Upledger discovered that many aspects of the work could be learned by patient and sensitive laypeople. This was the beginning of his making these skills available to a broader range of allied health care professionals and to family members of patients.

In the following years, many others have appeared who have had the skill and interest to make this therapy available. Thus, dedicated professionals from around the world and from many walks of life augment the teaching initiated by John Upledger and his staff.

Today craniosacral therapy is studied and practiced by massage therapists, dentists, physical therapists, and medical doctors. The developing study and practice of craniosacral therapy is greatly enriched by the qualities brought by this wide range of participants.

Though craniosacral therapy originated in the United States, it is now taught and practiced widely throughout North America and Europe. It has found a place in Japan, India, Australia, and many other countries.

What Is Craniosacral Therapy?

The term *craniosacral* refers to the practitioner's focus on the spinal column, the bones of the head or cranium, and the broad ending structure of the spine, the sacrum. As an evaluative and monitoring tool, craniosacral practice pays particular attention to the craniosacral rhythm, a slight swelling and contraction of the bones of the head, and a rotation around a central axis by the skeleton on each side of the body.

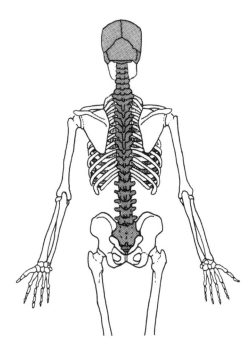

Figure 1. The Central Column: Sacrum, Spine, and Cranium. Within the human skeleton, the sacrum, spine, and cranium form a flexible central column. The entire column responds to the craniosacral rhythm and transmits this rhythm to the other bones and tissues of the body.

This regular movement is apparently generated by pressure changes throughout the head and spinal column during the production and absorption of cerebrospinal fluid. The craniosacral rhythm can be palpated throughout the human body at a rate of four to twelve cycles each minute. It offers a useful clue to the condition of soft tissue and joints throughout the body, and furnishes a diagram to patterns of pain and discomfort.

Yet, this important indicator of harmony or disharmony within the total being is barely utilized or even recognized by modern medical practitioners. As mentioned above, because the craniosacral rhythm is so subtle, difficulty in its perception serves as one of the main stumbling blocks to the vast realms opened by means of craniosacral practice. Patience and a degree of inner harmony are the most powerful keys to opening this realm for the new student.

Another important element of this practice is the fascia. All body parts are encased within a network of fibrous connective tissue. This varies from very thin, weblike film to many layers of specialized membranes. The most obvious of these is the cutaneous membrane, our outer skin. Internally, these varied protective membranes are called *fascias*.

A wonderful aspect of the body's fascia or connective tissue is that the entire network is interconnected and continuous. Thus, for example, the fascia surrounding the heart is connected and continuous with the fascia surrounding the lungs, arteries, nearby ribs and muscles, and, indirectly, with every other bodily organ.

The nerve material of the brain and spinal cord is covered on its surface by specialized fascia. This extends out onto the nerves and helps modulate nerve electrical qualities.

More important to our present interest is the inner lining of the skull and spinal column, especially the dura mater. This dense fibrous connective tissue lines the cranial vault, the bones surrounding the brain, and the nerve canal within the spinal column. This continuous sheath provides the chamber in which the cerebrospinal fluid circulates around the brain and spinal cord, from the top of the head to the end of the spine.

Together, the dura mater and the cerebrospinal fluid provide a cushioning and insulated environment for the important functions of the brain and spinal cord.

Yet, this protective membrane is itself vulnerable. As with any protective coating, the protective device itself can begin to collect evidence of stress. As a tent may begin to show wrinkles and sags while still protecting its occupants, so the dura mater, or any fascia, begins to show patterns of tightness and flexibility.

Within the human body, it appears that tension and strain patterns in the muscles and fibrous connective tissue are at the base of improper alignment of the bones. Prolonged tightness and inflexibility of the fascia or muscles creates a slight but steady pull on the bones, restricting movement and even shifting the bone from proper alignment. This is experienced as recurrent pain, propensity to repeated injury in the same place, and resistance to simple manipulative treatment. If a skilled practitioner realigns the bones themselves, relief may be temporary, because the connective tissues are transmitting to the bones a set of forces that gradually ease them out of alignment again. Craniosacral practice addresses the connective tissue more explicitly, eventually easing the internal stress and allowing the total system to rediscover a more harmonious alignment.

In the head, the dura mater is addressed, using a light touch on the cranial bones. In the trunk of the body, hands are applied in a number of crucial regions, called *diaphragms*. These are areas of the body where crosswise muscle and connective tissue predominate. Stress held in such tissue can contribute to misalignment or restriction. An obvious example is the respiratory diaphragm connecting across the lower ribs. Other diaphragms are located at the floor of the pelvis, across the shoulders, and at the point where the head and neck join.

Craniosacral practice is accomplished by careful attention to the rhythmic and energetic manifestations of the body. Gentle touch is applied in harmony with the indications received from the body, on the cranial bones and at the diaphragms. Craniosacral therapy originated within a tradition of physical manipulation. In some schools, strong pressures are still used for this work. Yet, the body often resists a forceful approach and responds readily to gentle touch. Essentially, this is a very simple therapy, a type of "laying on of hands," emanating from many years of sophisticated observation and experiment, and based on a profound attentiveness to and respect for the processes of the total person.

In craniosacral practice the craniosacral rhythm indicates symmetry, the bones serve as positioning devices for the therapist's hands, and muscle or connective tissue softens as physical harmony returns.

Benefits

The popularity of craniosacral therapy stems from its surprising versatility and effectiveness in treating injury and pain. Joints that have been impaired by injury or disease regain a wider range of motion. Shoulder, neck, and lower back pain are greatly eased through this work.

Persons suffering from chronic pain often enjoy relief and a new level of day-to-day functioning as a result of craniosacral treatments.

Frequently pain and injury present a pattern in a person's life. At times of stress, the same knee or hip flares up with pain after a small or unnoticed injury. Treatment often reveals that an original injury was suffered during a period of intense stress, anxiety, or confusion. The tendency to protectively tighten remains in the tissue and is aroused later under similar stress. This happens because body tissue has the capacity to "remember" injury and to be prepared to react more readily to similar injury at that point in the future. Unfortunately, the primary reaction of tissue to perceived trauma results in inflammation, swelling, stiffness and inflexibility of the affected area.

Unpleasant emotion, such as fear or anger, at the time of an injury seems to increase the severity of the protective reaction, prolong recovery, and increase the tissue's readiness to react protectively during a similar event in the future.

The gentle and supportive techniques of craniosacral treatments, which work with the tissue at the rate it is ready to respond, hold the key to releasing the tissue memory and the pattern of pain at that location.

The practitioner may use this work alone. Yet, as an effective complementary therapy, it facilitates other forms of treatment. For example, a chiropractic adjustment has often been found to be easier and to last longer after a craniosacral treatment. Craniosacral is used in conjunction with acupuncture, chiropractic, homeopathy, herbal remedies, psychotherapy, vision therapy, and traditional medicine.

Modern Practice

In recent years, chiropractors and physical therapists, massage therapists and psychotherapists, dentists and osteopaths have integrated this work into their healing efforts. They find that craniosacral therapy complements and enhances their more traditional forms of treatment. They notice more rapid and more profound results when craniosacral is applied together with conventional therapies to symptoms as varied as jaw pain, headaches, emotional crises, back, shoulder, or neck pain, and recurrent injuries. They have also found that craniosacral is a relaxing and regenerative treatment for almost anyone in our fast-paced world.

Craniosacral therapy is poised at the interface of conventional allopathic medicine and alternative modalities, which take a broader view of the human person, consciousness, suffering, and healing. The Age of

Reason and the age of modern science, mechanics, medicine, and philosophy turned resolutely away from any experience which could not be replicated in a mechanistic way and proven statistically. Anecdote, vision, intuition, and the spiritual were scorned by the "middle management," the bureaucrats of science. Our most creative thinkers, such as Einstein, transcended this bias. Otherwise, it has dominated formal education and research for many generations.

Today more and more investigators are regaining an appreciation of the broader capacities of the human being and considering the whole person in their treatment. The use of hypnosis, biofeedback, and even meditation to complement medical therapy at leading hospitals has stimulated the curiosity of many keen minds. These minds are now looking beyond the hard data of rigorous "scientific method" to the promising realm of possibility. The unifying theme in their efforts is the healing of the total person: physical, mental, and spiritual.

Part I

The Fundamentals of Craniosacral Therapy

The aim of this text is to communicate a basic understanding of craniosacral practice. This will involve evaluative skills: discovering the craniosacral rhythm and becoming sensitive to variations in the way the rhythm is transmitted throughout the body. It also involves a growing sense of how to take cues from variations in rhythm and from the many other energetic manifestations which act as nonverbal signals. This will be discussed in chapter 1.

The next step is learning how to use your hands to hold the tissue, follow its movement as it "unwinds," and make gentle adjustments in harmony with what we know of usual function at that place, and in harmony with what the tissue itself is ready to do. This will be discussed in chapters 2 and 3, dealing with the torso, then the head.

Finally, chapter 4 will discuss the attitude and wider context of craniosacral practice.

Many important physiological structures and functions will be described in this book. However, it is not comprehensive in its presentation of anatomy. It is helpful to have some knowledge or to consult an anatomy and physiology text. In particular, you may find it helpful to review skeletal structure, connective tissue, and the major pathways of the circulatory and nervous systems. An atlas of human anatomy will be useful to complement the illustrations and descriptions in this text.

Chapter 1

The Basic Skills for Craniosacral Practice

The craniosacral rhythm is a powerful yet subtle current that manifests the health of the protective environment of the brain and spinal cord. It provides clues regarding the alignment or misalignment of the bony structures of the head and extends its influence the length and width of the body. The craniosacral rhythm within the head and spinal cord appears to be produced by the cycle of production and absorption of cerebrospinal fluid. This takes place within the brain itself and within the protective covering of the dura mater.

The brain is a mass of specialized nerve cells, differentiated into sections by shape, by function, and by similarity to brains of other animals. The human brain contains nerve cells clustered into specialized sections which are similar in shape and function to the brains of other animals, with the addition of more highly elaborated brain sections possessed only by mammals.

The brain communicates with the total body through specialized nerve bundles that directly leave the brain to reach various organs, and by way of the spinal cord, which provides a protected conduit for thousands of pathways to every organ, sense receptor, muscle, or gland in the body.

Cerebrospinal fluid is produced within specially elaborated hollows, the ventricles, deep within the brain mass. The fluid is similar in physical characteristics and chemical composition to lymph or blood plasma. As it is produced, it passes from the series of ventricles within the brain to the spaces around the brain and spinal cord. This fluid is part of the protective and nurturing environment of the brain.

A tough membrane known as the dura mater adheres to the inner surface of the skull. Exiting at the foramen magnum, the dura forms a sleeve that extends downward within the spinal column. The spinal cord extends down this dural tube from the brain to its termination near the sacrum. Every fold and hollow of both brain and spinal cord is covered by a soft connective tissue known as the pia mater. Moreover, within the space between these membranes is an intermediary. Called the arachnoid membrane, it adheres to the inner surface of the dura and extends weblike fibers toward the pia mater. Cerebrospinal fluid flows within the space between membranes, that is, between arachnoid and pia mater.

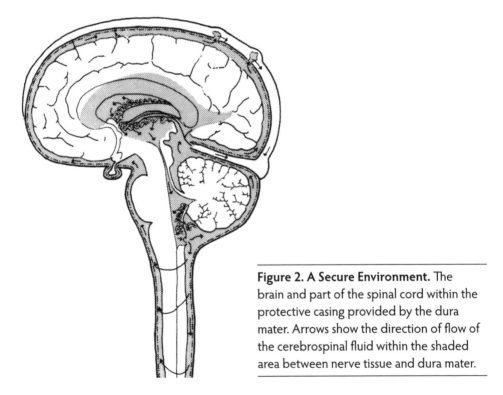

Figure 2. A Secure Environment. The brain and part of the spinal cord within the protective casing provided by the dura mater. Arrows show the direction of flow of the cerebrospinal fluid within the shaded area between nerve tissue and dura mater.

Cerebrospinal fluid flows within the spinal canal, down the back of the spinal cord and up the front, to bathe and cushion the outer surface of the brain. It is absorbed into the venous blood by specialized tissue in the fascia that protrudes into the venous blood vessels (the arachnoid villi).

Thus a living source of nutrients and protection surrounds and bathes the core of the human nervous system. It is constantly flowing and renewing itself. The mechanism of this renewal produces the craniosacral rhythm. As fluid is secreted by specialized tissue in the ventricles, pressure within the entire cerebrospinal system increases. As the bones of the cranial vault spread to accommodate this pressure, the changes are monitored by sense receptors in the cranial sutures, the joints between skull bones. A signal is sent from receptor to brain, and secretion of fluid is halted. As absorption progresses, system pressure reduces until resumption of secretion is signaled. The cycle begins anew.

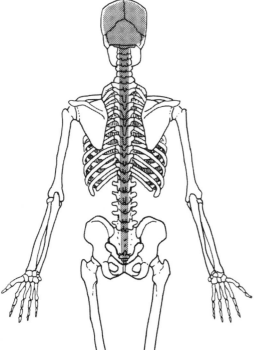

Figure 3. Fluid Circulation. Cerebrospinal fluid circulates within the shaded area shown here. It flows from the cranial vault through the spinal canal to the sacrum, and returns to be absorbed within the cranial vault.

Changes in pressure within the cranial vault and the spinal column result in skeletal shifts through the structure of spine and cranium. These can be palpated in all the bones of the head and face, and at the end of the spine at the sacrum.

Through a mechanism that is not clearly understood, the paired bones on each side of the central column also respond to these pressure changes. The shoulders, ribs, hips, and legs move in unison with the craniosacral rhythm.

These movements provide keys to the condition of the fascia or soft tissue of the body, and to the flexibility of the joints throughout head and body. If joints have become impacted, the asymmetric or constricted movement can be felt. If muscle or fascia is chronically tight, then symmetrical movement of the spine is impaired and can be palpated. Thus, perception of the craniosacral rhythm is a valuable aid in healing or releasing patterns of restriction and pain.

Perceiving the Craniosacral Rhythm

A series of exercises can help in becoming attuned to the craniosacral rhythm. They involve sense awareness of the perceptible rhythms of the body: heart, breath, and craniosacral. We will describe and experiment with them.

A helpful attitude toward the following explorations might combine curiosity and playfulness.

Even if you are experienced in taking pulse or monitoring respiration, I urge you to perform these exercises. They form an introduction to the attitudes of respect, awareness, and active receptivity that are important components of craniosacral assessment and treatment.

The exercises are in the form of guided meditations. As you read or listen to them, you can set aside or ignore, for the time, the business of the logical mind. Let yourself sink into these explorations, into a different dimension of experience. Let yourself trust, for the time, without judgment, your perceptions or intuitions.

Some people may find it helpful to tape these exercises. If you do so, speak slowly and deliberately, pausing between phrases. Then sit quietly and listen, following the guidance of your own voice. Allow an interval between exercises.

I suggest that these exercises be practiced in a chair, sitting comfortably but straight, hands resting on your thighs, arms and shoulders loose.

Exercise 1: The Heart

Sitting quietly ... feeling hands on thighs ... feeling
    the pressure of the chair against your body ...

Feeling easy ... breathing easily ... relaxed ...

Aware of your body ... aware of the heartbeat ... somewhere in
    your body ... your heartbeat ... your body ...

Sinking into this exploration ... tuning in ... to feelings ...
    energies ... to your heartbeat ...

Imagine the location of your heart.... Do you feel its action
    there?... In the center of your chest?... At the sides?

Wherever you sense, feel, imagine the heartbeat,...
    it continues ... unnoticed ... noticed ...

Imagine where you would feel the pulse on your wrist....
    Without touching with your fingers,... what do you sense
    in your wrist?... As the pulse continues ...

In your hands ... arms ...

Can you feel the heartbeat in your throat?

Your face ...

Is there a sensation of heartbeat in your feet?... your calves?...
    your thighs?...

Moving from place to place in your body ... feeling
the heart pulsation ... feeling how it is different ... from place
to place ...

Enjoying this exploration ... refreshed and at ease ... sitting
quietly ... feeling the pressure of the chair ...

Preparing to return to ordinary awareness ... your heart
pulsation continues ... noticed ... unnoticed ... as you bring
your attention to other occupations ... other interests ...

Becoming aware of your surroundings ... feeling like stretching ...
or moving ... looking around ... fully returning to your usual
awareness.

Take as much time as you wish with this exercise. When you repeat it
later, you may enjoy noticing how you devise your own elaboration.

Exercise 2: The Breath

Sitting quietly ... feeling hands on thighs ... feeling
the pressure of the chair against your body ...

Feeling easy ... breathing easily ... relaxed ...

Aware of your body ... aware of your breathing ...
your chest moving ...

Feeling the breath in your nostrils ... in your throat ...
in the whole body ...

Allowing eyes to close ... as you continue ... breathing ...
feeling the breath ...

Feeling the difference ... of closing eyes ... changing perception ...
awareness ... of breath in nostrils ...
in throat ... in chest ...

Breathing fully ... easily ...

Lifting chest ... lifting shoulders ... with each breath ... moving
the body ... continuing ...

Feeling the breath pressing on belly ... or sides ...

How do you feel the breath in your pelvis?... breathing
fully ... breathing easily ...

Is there any effect of your breath on your legs?... your thighs?...

Letting your wrists and hands rest lightly on your thighs,... how
do you perceive the movement of your breath in your upper
arms?...

What do you notice in your elbows?... wrists?... hands?...

Do your hands perceive any motion in your thighs?...

Do you have any wish to use your hands to explore
the sensation of heart and lungs on your body?... exploring
the motion of body with breath ...

Have you noticed your heartbeat, superimposed on each breath?...

How far you can follow this heartbeat ... superimposed
on breath ...

In chest ... belly ... in your neck ... your face ...

And notice how much you enjoy this time, this opening
of awareness to your body and its rhythms ...

Notice, also, how you may have branched out on your own
explorations, or developed your own rate of inquiry ...

You may realize that with each exercise you have broadened
your sensitivity ... allowed an experience that will remain
with you ...

As you prepare to return to your ordinary awareness …
to bring your attention to other occupations and interests …

Refreshed … intrigued … by this experience …

Eyes opening … moving … stretching … looking … fully
returning to your usual awareness.

Exercise 3: The Craniosacral Rhythm: Awareness

Sitting quietly … feeling hands on thighs … feeling
the pressure of the chair against your body …

Feeling easy … breathing easily … relaxed …

Aware of your body … aware of arms … legs … back … neck …

Eyes open … or closing … breathing …

Sinking … into a new exploration … of body … of awareness …

Cerebrospinal fluid is produced … as I breathe … sitting here …

Produced … and absorbed …

Cerebrospinal fluid is produced … as I sit here … my cranial
bones expanding … at the sutures … and returning …

Cerebrospinal fluid produced … and absorbed …

The bones in my head … adjusting … the cranial vault
expanding … and returning …

Expanding … and returning … as cerebrospinal fluid
is produced … and absorbed …

My shoulders rotate backward … with each expansion …
and return forward …

Rotating backward … and returning forward …

Shoulders ... and ribs ... rotating ... and returning ...
with each cycle ...

As I continue ... breathing ... adjusting ... in my body ...
in the bones of my head ... to each cycle ... in the
craniosacral rhythm ...

Cerebrospinal fluid produced ... and flowing ... within
the cranium ... within the spine ...

Cerebrospinal fluid ... flowing ... produced ... and absorbed ... each
cycle ... the cranial vault expanding outward ...
and returning inward ... each cycle ...

Shoulders and ribs ... rotating backward ... and returning ...
shoulders ... ribs ... even hips ... rotating ... and returning ...
each cycle ...

The tissue and fascia accommodating ... adjusting ... to each
expansion ... to each return ...

To each rotation ... and return ...

The tissue ... the fascia ...

As I breathe inward ... my shoulders lift slightly ... and return ...

As cerebrospinal fluid is produced ... my shoulders rotate
slightly ... and return ... rotate ... and return ... at each cycle
of the craniosacral rhythm ...

As my hands and wrists rest on my thighs,... have I discovered
yet ... their motion?...

Rotating outward ... and returning ...

Outward ... and returning inward ...

My hands on my thighs ... moving with the craniosacral rhythm ...

All the tissue … all the cells … responding … adjusting …
   to this rhythm … expanding … returning …

My feet responding … my legs … my shoulders …
   unnoticed … noticed … continuing …

Breathing … with this rhythm … discovering … rediscovering …

The rhythm … the heartbeat … the breath … the craniosacral
   rhythm …

Relaxing … at ease … playing … discovering …

Ready soon to return … to ordinary awareness … returning with
   new awareness … new wondering …

Sitting … aware of the pressure of the chair against my body …

Returning refreshed … remembering other occupations
   and interests …

To my surroundings … to ordinary awareness … moving …
   stretching … looking.

Exercise 4: The Craniosacral Rhythm: Palpation

For this exercise, sit at a table. Support your elbows on the
   table, so that you can lightly touch the upper sides of your
   head with your fingers. A book or two under your elbows
   may help to position your hands. Arrange yourself so your
   shoulders, neck, and head are supported as usual by your
   spinal column, rather than by your hands or arms.

Sitting quietly … feeling hands on the side of the head … arms
   and elbows supported …

Feeling the pressure of the chair … supporting the body …

Breathing freely … and easily …

Aware of your heartbeat ... sensations of fingers contacting
 scalp ... warmth ... coolness ...

Heartbeat ... breath ...

Fingertips ... fingers ... moving with scalp ... moving with the
 craniosacral rhythm ...

Head bones moving ... expanding outward ... returning inward ...

Expanding outward ... returning inward ...

With each cycle of the craniosacral rhythm ... with each cycle of
 cerebrospinal fluid ... produced ... absorbed ...

A regular rhythm ... soft ... subtle ... outward ... inward ...

Breathing freely ... deeply or lightly ... breathing freely ...
 deeply or lightly ... discovering ...

Holding the breath ... noticing ... sensing ... releasing the
 breath ... breathing easily ... freely ...

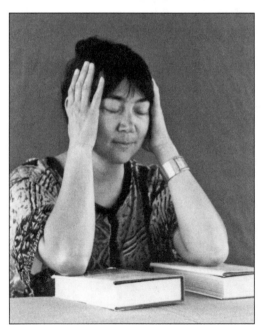

Figure 4. Palpation of the Craniosacral Rhythm on Oneself. Hands softly on sides of head; head supported by neck and spine.

Hands and fingers ... touching ... sensing ... moving in
harmony with the rhythm ... outward ... inward ...

Inward ... outward ... the cerebrospinal fluid ... produced ...
absorbed ...

A movement ... a rhythm ... that can pause ... inward or
outward ... can pause ... become still ...

Sinking in ... recognizing ... experiencing ... the craniosacral
rhythm ...

Continuing ... the rhythm ... of learning ... of experience ...
and discovery ...

The rhythm ... full ... regular ...

Movement in hands ... in cranial vault ...

Aware of rhythm ... aware of body ... of body energy ... feet ...
arms ... the whole body ...

Preparing to return ... to ordinary awareness ... sitting ... hands
on sides of head ... chair ... the room ...

Returning fully to ordinary awareness ... to other occupations
and interests ...

Alert ... aware and curious ... as you complete this exercise.

It will be helpful for you to repeat this exercise more than once. I would
recommend that you vary it with the preceding exercises. Between times
get up, move around, stretch, sing, dance, or whatever appeals to you.

As you return to these exercises, return refreshed, with a new perspective. The craniosacral rhythm is strong, enduring, unfailing except for
points of stillness. Yet, it is subtle. And the more refreshed the mind and
body, the greater ease in perceiving it.

When you have begun to perceive the craniosacral rhythm, continue some form of these exercises as a means to go deeper, to absorb more.

Listening Stations

We will now go through a series of listening stations. At each, you will have the opportunity to perceive and assess the craniosacral rhythm. Perception of that rhythmic movement distinguishes this work from other forms of therapy. Yet, the impulses known as the craniosacral rhythm are not the only signals manifested by the client in this interactive procedure. Each one of us brings to this work special qualities and skills of observation and awareness. These nonverbal skills often lie dormant as we adapt to modern technological society. This work furnishes an opportunity to reawaken these fundamental perceptual capacities. Thus you may sense variations in warmth, flow, breathing, or skin coloring. You may also sense energetic qualities. Any of these qualities have an equally important place with the craniosacral rhythm.

The listening stations are

1. the feet

2. the thighs

3. the hips

4. the respiratory diaphragm

5. the shoulders

6. the head

Later, these procedures become part of the assessment phase of a craniosacral session. For now, please consider these to be exercises, which you will repeat frequently, gaining valuable knowledge and experience each time. If you imagine you feel the rhythm or something like the rhythm, assume that you do. The strength of the craniosacral rhythm varies from person to person, and among listening stations on the same person.

After a few minutes at each station, allow yourself to move on, gaining a broad experience, even when you are not sure what you feel at first. Repetition of these experiences will result in growing familiarity and confidence in your perceptions. There is a vast realm of experience and insight ahead of you.

The explorations in this section are accomplished most easily with a partner, whom we will call your client. It is best to work on a clear table, 28 to 30 inches (70 to 76 centimeters) above the floor. A massage table is excellent, but any strong table covered with a soft pad will do. Have a chair or stool available that can be easily moved around the table and that allows you to sit with your knees and legs under the table. A few cushions to adjust the height will also be useful. An adjustable secretarial chair is very useful.

For most craniosacral work, the client can wear lightweight, loose clothing. It is helpful to remove jewelry, watches, belts, or anything that binds or provides bulk. For warmth, a blanket can be used, and moved aside as you work.

Ask your client to lie on the table, face upward. As part of a standard procedure, ensure that your client is comfortable. A pillow or bolster may be inserted under the knees later, as the session progresses. This is especially helpful in easing stress on the lower back.

If your client is pregnant, she may be more comfortable on her side, with a pillow between her knees, and another pillow to hold at her chest. As therapist, you can learn to adapt to this position in your work.

Terminology

These exercises, and the instructions throughout this book, often refer to directions such as higher, lower, front and back, posterior, anterior, inward, outward. These are in relation to the client's body, with the direction of the head being upward or *superior,* and the direction of the feet being downward or *inferior.*

Anterior refers to the front or a movement to the front of the body; *posterior* refers to the back or a movement toward the back.

Inward and *outward* are used interchangeably with the anatomical directions, *medial* and *lateral,* to refer to horizontal movement between the centerline and the side of the body.

For example, if your hand is on the client's hip, and you move it to the ribs, you are moving upward or superiorly on the client's body. If you move your hand or attention from the client's back to his or her front, as the client is lying on the table, you are moving anteriorly or forward (not upward).

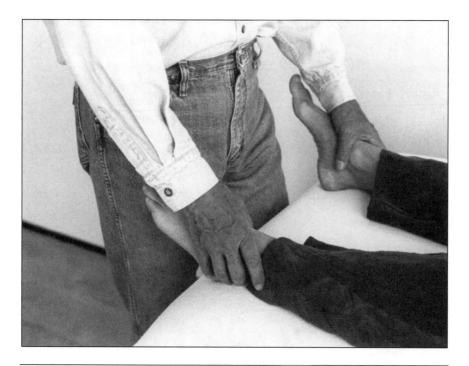

Figure 5. Listening Station at the Feet. Lightly grasping the ankles.

Self-awareness

Throughout these exercises, you are reminded to assess and respond to your own physical state as well as the client's. The entire procedure is interactive. Your consideration and concern for your own comfort and energy flow is an important aspect of the total treatment situation.

1. Feet

Stand at the client's feet, and let your hands lightly grasp the ankles and upper feet from the front. Continue to breathe comfortably and easily. If you are leaning forward expectantly, move your body gently to relax your muscles. Bring your energy back from your hands so that your touch is light, physically and energetically.

What do you feel? A pulse, a slight movement with the client's breathing, warmth or coolness? As you become aware of the craniosacral rhythm you will sense a slight rotation outward and inward, similar to what you have experienced in your own thighs and shoulders.

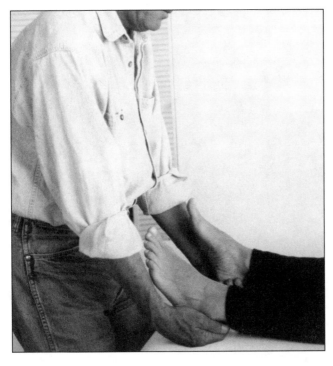

Figure 6. Listening Station at the Feet. Hands supporting the heels.

In many clients, you will notice a difference from one foot to the other in the rotation produced by the craniosacral rhythm. You may perceive pauses or differences of tempo during each cycle of movement.

Note the tension or relaxation in your own hands, arms, shoulders, or any other part of your body. Experiment with your stance and breathing. How can you be physically at ease while remaining attuned to the client and maintaining only a light touch?

Allow your attention to go back and forth from your own body to the client. Adjust your grasp: it should be firm but light.

After only a few minutes, release your grasp and move your hands under the heels, grasping fully and lightly. Repeat your inquiries here as before. Differences from front to back at the ankles often reflect conditions of ease and restriction, front and back, in the pelvis.

Again, after a few minutes, gently release your contact as you prepare to move to the next station.

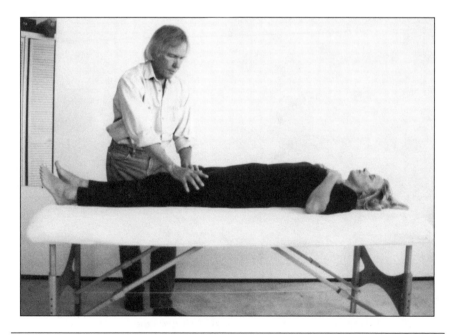

Figure 7. Listening Station at the Upper Leg. Hands resting on the thighs.

2. Thighs

Now, go to one side of the table so that you can rest your hands on the client's thighs. Let your hands conform to the contour of the body at this location, using a light touch along the whole contact surface. How can you position your body so that you are most at ease as you do this?

As you stand, making contact, can you visualize a sphere of energy that includes both you and your client? Within this ambiance, attune yourself to energy and movement.

What do you perceive at this station? Heartbeat, warmth, motion of breathing, craniosacral motion … Do the thighs move in unison as they rotate outward and inward? Do you have a sense of energy flow lengthwise through the area? Do you sense pockets of more intense energy in the pelvis or hips as you observe from this position?

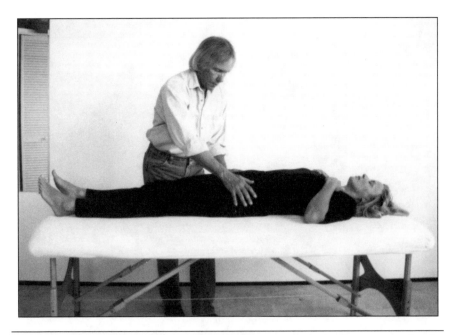

Figure 8. Listening Station at the Hips. Hands resting on the hip bones on each side.

Do the variations in the craniosacral rhythm remind you of those you experienced at the client's feet?

After a few minutes, release your contact and prepare to move to the next station. At this point, your client may be made more comfortable by placing a support such as a pillow under the knees, lifting them and easing the lower back.

3. Hips

Position yourself beside the client, slightly below the pelvis, so that you can place your hands on the forward edge of the hip bones. Experiment with your posture and hand placement so that your hands are in contact with the front edge and side of each hip bone.

The craniosacral rhythm at this location causes the bones under your hands to rotate inward and outward around the center of the body. Because of the many directions of force from the skeleton and muscles in this region, the pelvis is very vulnerable to restrictions of movement and foci or cysts of energy. As you palpate the rhythm, note the differences between the sides in the completion of the cycle, as well as any differences in smoothness of the cycle from one side to the other.

Be aware of any sensation of energy intensity that you may experience in the pelvic area. Your attention may even be drawn to places you are not directly contacting.

As an experiment, attempt to visualize the juncture of the hip with each side of the sacrum. Imagine the movement in these joints, in coordination with the movement you feel under your hands. Do you sense any areas of energy or lack of energy in this whole area?

After a few minutes, withdraw your contact so that you can move to the following station.

4. Respiratory Diaphragm

At this station, place your hands at each side on the client's lower ribs, conforming your contact to the body contour. Reassure the client that it is all right to continue breathing naturally.

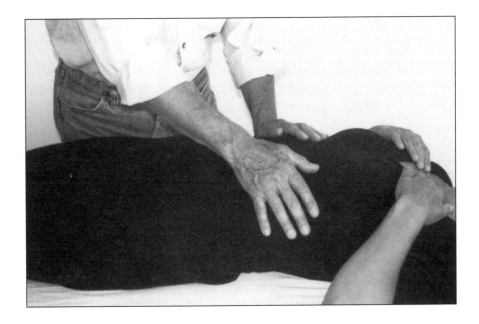

Figure 9. Listening Station at the Respiratory Diaphragm.
Hands on each side resting on the lower ribs.

This is a very challenging place to discover the craniosacral rhythm. Let yourself be at ease and breathing naturally, too. Visualize the sphere of energy including both you and your client. Within that sphere, you can be open to any movement, physiological or energetic.

You will notice the heartbeat and the motions of breathing. What other motions or energies do you sense? The craniosacral rhythm produces a motion of the ribs, spreading outward and returning inward, against the backdrop of the rising and falling abdomen and chest. It is usually a little slower than the rhythm of the breath.

When I first sensed the craniosacral rhythm in these circumstances, it was very exciting. But there is no urgency. You are gathering considerable information already, both at a conscious and a nonconscious level. Observe whatever information is available: energy movement or concentration; warmth or coolness; variations in the movement from side to side.

Within a few minutes, withdraw your contact and prepare to move to the next station.

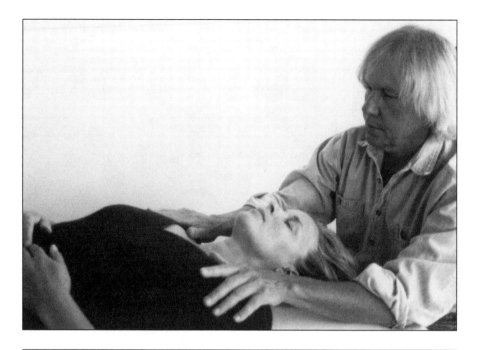

Figure 10. Listening Station at the Shoulders. Hands on each side, resting on the shoulders and upper chest.

5. Shoulders

Now move to the end of the table, at the client's head. Sit on a chair, resting your elbows on the table. Place your palms on each side, contacting the client's shoulders and upper chest. Allow some time to become comfortable and acquainted with the various components of movement you experience.

Let your hands conform to the body contours: stay in contact, yet keep it light. Your hands are most effective when the touch is light and responsive to motion in any dimension. Assess the sensations in your own shoulders and arms. Are you at ease? Breathing freely?

The heartbeat provides a steady pulsation throughout the chest. Again, the motion of breathing dominates at this station. The breath tends to lift the chest forward and outward from the body. It may draw the shoulders upward, toward the ears. The craniosacral rhythm can be identified because it lifts the shoulders directly upward from the table, moving in an arc around the vertical centerline of the body.

Again, do not be discouraged if you do not perceive the craniosacral rhythm in your first efforts at palpation. At some level you are learning, aware, and in contact.

After a few minutes release your contact and draw back slightly. Bring your awareness to the client's neck and head.

6. Head (Cranium)

As you touch the head, it is important to be able to rest your forearms on the table. Feel free to ask your client to move downward so there is a space of 6 or 8 inches (18 to 24 centimeters) above the head. As you work with the neck and head, maintain your awareness of the entire interconnected structure. As you place your hands, lift, or move the head, be sensitive to the fluidity or resistance you experience. At this stage, keep the head

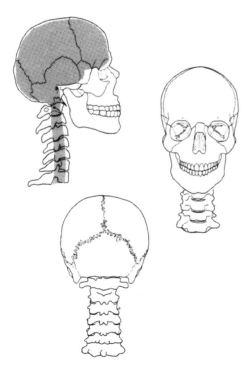

Figure 11. The Structure of the Head and Neck. Shading in the side view depicts the position of the brain and spinal cord within the protective bony structure. Lines on the skull indicate sutures or joints between bones.

and neck aligned with the spine, but do not force the alignment. In any movement, go with the direction of ease.

a.) Place your hands, palms upward, on each side of the client's head. Slide them under the skull, toward each other, and cradle the back and sides of the head. (See figure 12.) Adjust your hands so that they are comfortable to you, the therapist, and to your client. Your forearms will be resting on the table, but keep them loose, rather than supporting your weight. Breathe easily and observe the sensations in your own shoulders and neck as you work.

As you attune yourself to the sensations in your hands, you may observe a slight pulling of the client's head and neck toward the body with each inhalation. Accustom yourself to that.

Have you noticed a heartbeat? Yours? Your client's?

The craniosacral rhythm may be experienced as a slight outward swelling of the skull, and a return inward. You may sense it as skull move-

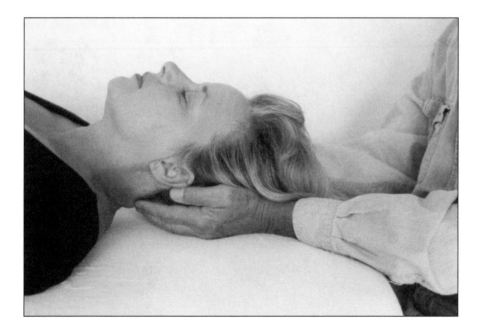

Figure 12. Listening Station at the Head: a.) Hands cradling the back and sides of the head.

ment. Or you may notice your hands moving rhythmically inward and outward.

The rhythm may be quite harmonious at this location. Or you may feel that one side seems to swell more fully than the other, or that the rhythm seems to push outward more than inward, or inward more than outward. You may sense energy, warmth, even a feeling of electricity.

Allow yourself to observe the rhythm and any variations for a few minutes. Then prepare to change your hand position.

b.) Slide one hand completely under the back of your client's head. Help lift and stabilize the head with your other hand. When you feel secure with the weight of the head in the palm of one hand, bring your other hand upward and lay it across the top of the head, overlapping your fingers onto the forehead. (See figure 13.) Allow full contact with your fingers and palm. Yet, this is only a touch, not a pressure.

Some people are sensitive to touch on the forehead. Often, the difficulty is not the pressure, but the energetic intensity of the therapist. After

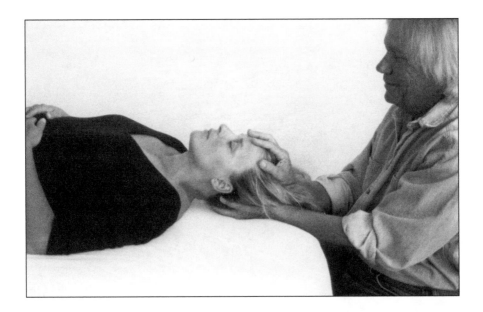

Figure 13. Listening Station at the Head: b.) One hand supporting the head, fingers of the other hand lightly resting on the forehead.

making contact, sink back physically and energetically. Maintaining touch, notice the feel of your feet on the floor or the chair supporting you. This tends to balance your energy so that it is not so concentrated. The lighter the touch and the less the effort, the more that you will feel.

The main component of the craniosacral rhythm is a swelling forward (anteriorly) of the forehead, and a return. You may notice a greater range on one side or the other, or be more aware of the rhythm on one side of the cycle, either inward or outward. At times, therapists have observed a twisting motion of the frontal bone (forehead) during the cycle of the craniosacral rhythm. Any movement or rhythm that you notice is the correct thing to notice, even if it does not conform to an idealized description of the craniosacral rhythm.

After a few moments, release the head by bringing your hand off the top of the head and using it for support and stability as you disengage both hands. Use this transition time to assess your own state of harmony and ease. Move or stretch if it helps you to be more present.

c.) When you are ready, bring your hands to each side of the client's head, so that the pad of the thumb rests lightly at each temple. (See figure

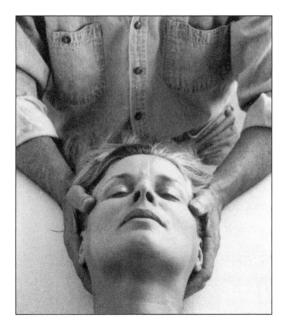

Figure 14. Listening Station at the Head: c.) Hands on each side of the head; thumbs at the temples, at the greater wings of the sphenoid.

14.) On each side, the thumb contact is just behind the corner of the eye. Let the hands and other fingers touch softly where they reach comfortably. Be at ease. Let any tension in your hands, arms, and shoulders drain to the floor.

You will not directly feel bone here. Rather, many muscle attachments originate here and extend down to the lower jaw, passing under the zygomatic arch (the prominent ridge extending forward from the ears).

Beneath the pads of your thumbs, covered by muscle, are the broad extensions of the sphenoid bone. The sphenoid forms the base of the cranial vault, that is, the base of the bony structure that protects the brain. The sphenoid forms a joint with each of the other bones enclosing the brain. It also touches directly or indirectly the bones of the face and mouth. Many nerves and blood vessels pass through small openings in the sphenoid to the eyes, face, and jaw. Free and balanced movement of the sphenoid is important to harmonious functioning and flow within the face and its organs.

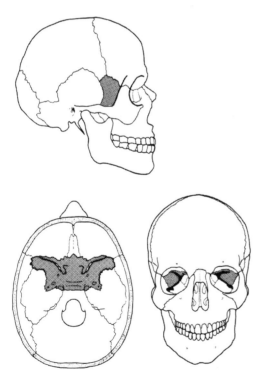

Figure 15. The Sphenoid. Three views of the sphenoid bone in relation to the rest of the skull. The cutaway view at bottom left looks into the skull from above. It shows how the sphenoid articulates with every other cranial bone, as it forms the inner floor of the cranial vault. The "wings" on each side curve upward at the temples, behind the eye sockets, providing a surface to sense and follow the motion of the bone.

What are you sensing with your hands? Components of breath and heartbeat? Warmth or coolness? Have you noticed the swelling outward and return of the skull?

When you notice the motion of the greater wings of the sphenoid, it will appear to move the pads of your thumbs inferiorly, toward the jaw, and superiorly, toward the top of the head. Notice if the rhythm is stronger in one direction or the other, or uneven from side to side. Be aware of the lightness of your touch. Ask your client if the position is comfortable.

After a few minutes, disengage and move away from your client. When you have been so intimately in contact, it is helpful to move away slowly.

It is also important to disengage completely, allowing individual space for each of you. Take a few moments to return to your more ordinary level of awareness. Move and stretch. Breathe! Encourage your client to do the same, as he or she is ready.

We have now completed the listening stations.

When you and your client share your experiences with each other, it is not unusual to discover that each has felt different components of the same thing: each experiences the movement or energy from a different perspective. Sharing can broaden your view of what occurred, and each viewpoint is valid.

Repeat these listening station exercises. If possible, use a variety of clients. You will notice differences between clients: age differences (e.g., age twenty and age forty); differences in strength of craniosacral rhythm; patterns of differences from side to side. You will grow in confidence and capability in perceiving the craniosacral rhythm, and in perceiving other patterns of energy restriction and flow.

Assessment, Awareness

The listening stations serve as an introduction to the assessment process in a craniosacral session.

Assessment in craniosacral practice does not mean formulating a diagnosis and a specific set of treatment procedures. Rather, assessment means employing a set of skills involving awareness and touch throughout the session. The information gained directs and redirects each step of the treatment session. On a larger scale, this is true of any therapeutic regime. The unique aspect here is that the practitioner observes and responds to changes during a treatment session.

It becomes apparent that every component and position on the client's body is related to every other component or position. A modification in tissue tone or energy at one point results in changes in other locations, also. A release of constriction or pain may allow the emergence of an older, underlying pattern of trauma that was not evident at the onset of treatment.

Assessment indicates to the practitioner whether to remain longer at this location, or move on. Assessment always continues hand in hand with the treatment procedure, minute to minute, in the here and now.

Yet, for now there is no need to draw detailed conclusions from your listening stations with each client. Rather, you are building up a body of experience and skill. This will be increased greatly, and have more meaning, as you practice the therapeutic releases described in the next two chapters.

The experience and skill you are developing includes components that go far beyond a set of techniques. As you gain experience and progress, you will find yourself developing a sensitivity and awareness that extends beyond ordinary waking conscious awareness and logical analysis. This sensitivity and awareness encompasses both yourself and your client and is crucial for accessing the full capabilities of craniosacral practice. The exercises designed for this book aim to assist you in developing the fullest level of skill in all these dimensions. That is why you are encouraged to practice the exercises, or develop similar ones for yourself, even if you are already familiar with some of the skills described.

Awareness

In ordinary day-to-day experience, our conscious awareness is mostly focused on the mechanics of living: traveling to work, running errands, keeping up with the news, managing time and money. Most people are aware we also function in other dimensions than the ordinarily conscious. Crucial bodily functions operate without conscious awareness or direction. At times these bodily functions can be influenced positively through interaction with our conscious awareness. For example, meditation has been shown to help reduce high blood pressure. Hypnosis has been found to help improve memory and learning, relieve pain, control bleeding during surgery, and hasten healing after surgery.

Ordinary conscious awareness can be specialized for each individual. Some people are more conscious of color, some of form. Some are very alert to practical considerations and the way things work mechanically. Others more easily see connections and possibilities of design and decor. Some people are considered more sensitive or intuitive because they more readily perceive and respond to social or emotional nuances. Their ordinary conscious awareness has capabilities that are obvious, though not well understood.

This book aims to recognize and accept the unique conscious base that each individual has to offer and to help expand the capability of that conscious awareness into new dimensions.

Some of these dimensions will be technical: understanding structure, functions, and relationships in the human body; understanding important aspects of working as a therapist with another person. Some dimensions will be more intuitive: a capability for responding to energetic signals with appropriate movements and pressures; an awareness of self that keeps pace with the developing awareness of the client.

Touch

There is an important reason for developing this broader awareness of yourself and your touch. Just as lovers may respond to each other intuitively with great sensitivity, so the hands of therapists often touch the "right" place without thought. I have observed the hands of beginning practitioners moving in harmony with the client's rhythm or tissue release while the practitioner is distractedly wondering what technique to use next.

As you develop a broader awareness of your subtle body movements and sensations, your interaction with your client will become your chief teacher. You will learn to follow your intuition, to follow your hands.

There is a touch which is a habit: grasping a friend's arm or hand; standing close or far away while conversing; using firm touch or light touch; stroking one's chin; rubbing one's face. There are touches that combine habit and technique: a massage therapist completing a routine that has been repeated many times; a pianist playing a familiar piece while preoccupied with a personal problem.

The goal here is to suspend habit for the time of the session so that the therapist-client interaction is truly present here and now, combining intuition with past learning and experience.

Understanding the Organism as a Whole

A hallmark of alternative health care is the effort to understand and cope with the organism as a totality. A special weakness of conventional medicine is its occupation with specific symptoms. All too often in our fast-paced society a client wants to merely alleviate the symptom so he or she can return to life as usual. We now understand that this approach merely buries the underlying problem that the symptom is expressing.

For instance, during times of stress, one person is likely to catch a cold, while another might come down with the flu. Someone else might be vulnerable to sleeplessness or a flare-up of recurrent back pain. Conventional medicine provides substances that reduce pain, inhibit mucus production, induce sleep, or relax muscles.

With these medications a person can push onward, continuing a stressful lifestyle, building up a large debt to self in terms of propensity to aches and pains and susceptibility to disease, and ultimately inviting a more rapid breakdown of body functions with advancing age. A frequent comment made by those who have disregarded the messages of the body: "I don't understand. I used to be able to do this with no problem."

Each illness, ache, or pain is a nonverbal message from the cellular or organ level to conscious awareness: pay attention, be aware of what you're doing to yourself. It is usually after prolonged stress or repeated injury that a seriously confining illness or disability occurs. Merely treating the most inflamed or restricted area fails to address the total constellation of traumatized tissue with its propensity to injury or illness. For more comprehensive healing to occur, the therapist looks at all the information being presented by the body and teaches the client to do the same.

Another approach to illness or injury has been to ask, is this physical or psychological? This is not a helpful question. It is based on our wish to have a clear, simple answer to disturbing questions.

Human existence is more complex than that. We can differentiate physiological, emotional, mental, and spiritual aspects of a person. Yet we are one, a unity. Every movement, every accident, every joy or discovery occurs within us in our totality. Every headache, backache, or illness is physical *and* psychological, and also spiritual, as well as any other aspect we are capable of differentiating. Comprehensive healing occurs when practitioner and client are open to information from the whole person.

The attitude of the therapist in assessment is that of attentiveness, of openness, even of curiosity. Curiosity admits that it does not know the whole story yet, and is eager to discover what is happening here. On the individual level, there is truly not a set answer as to how a problem was caused or how to treat it.

The fact that there are not simple answers is not a difficulty, but part of the adventure in a healing practice. If an attitude of openness and experimentation is kept, the body itself will indicate how to proceed, and what has priority.

Again, respect, awareness, and openness in listening are key. These are qualities that are embedded throughout this book. In chapter 4 we will return to the topic of assessment, building on the experience you have gained in performing a full craniosacral session.

Chapter 2

Releasing the Body

The listening stations provide a beginning framework for touch and mutual awareness in a craniosacral session. As you moved along, you were encouraged to be aware of any of the various signals emanating from the body tissue: the craniosacral rhythm and any other motion or energy you perceived. Now we will work more intensively at a number of positions along the torso and neck while maintaining this attitude of broad awareness, mutual respect, and curiosity.

Therapeutic Release

Release is simply the easing of constriction in muscle and connective tissue. Release of constriction allows the body to reestablish a more natural balance among its parts. It results in an easing of pressure on joints. Release allows a healthy flow of nerve impulse, fluid, and energy between regions of the body.

A therapeutic release occurs when tissue that has held the imprint of a past injury or affliction releases that imprint, freeing itself for a fuller and more ordinary range of functioning. *Tissue memory* is a term that has been devised to explain a set of experiences and suppositions by therapists. Certain injuries recur even after they appear to have healed; common examples are injuries to the back, neck, or jaw. Certain illnesses tend to recur—some people have colds more than others, some have headaches, others are prone to stomach ailments. Both injuries and illnesses tend to occur more frequently during periods of life stress. Physical exhaustion also seems to trigger chronic patterns of constriction or illness. The affliction is not random but specific to the individual.

Emotions are often associated with the lingering effects of illness or injury. Individuals differ in whether they feel calm or agitated, hopeless or hopeful when ill or in pain. During bodywork, as a pattern of pain or dysfunction eases, individuals sometimes experience a memory or strong emotion similar to that experienced when the injury or illness first occurred. Being touched in a specific place, such as the neck or leg, or finding the body in a certain position can trigger the memory and emotion.

Here is an example. While rotating among fellow students at a craniosacral training, I found myself working with a woman, holding her sacrum in one hand and the back of her head in the other. She began to feel upset and then to vividly recall an auto accident a year or more in the past. She was puzzled, because she had healed well from head and face injuries and apparently had left it all behind her. Nevertheless, as she experienced the emotions of the accident again a forgotten aspect emerged. At the moment of impact, her child screamed. As the woman was propelled forward and injured, she felt helpless and extremely worried for her child. As it turned out, her child was not injured, and during recovery that part of her own experience was forgotten. This brief intervention during a training session allowed her to go back to that moment and release a feeling of anxiety and helplessness that somehow had lingered below the level of conscious awareness.

How does the tissue hold the imprint of past experience? Although this is not fully understood, there are many mechanisms by which the body "learns" or adapts, based on experience. One is the operation of the immune system. When a foreign substance invades body tissue, a complex set of changes occurs in the blood, endocrine, and lymph systems. Specific substances are modified to neutralize the effect of the foreign substance. In addition, the body produces other substances that will be held in waiting so that the body can react more rapidly if a similar threat appears in the future.

Another mechanism acts at the nerve endings. When a particular set of stimuli are affecting a nerve ending, chemical substances are produced that will prepare the nerve to react more quickly when similar conditions recur.

These examples do not fully explain the complicated experience of tissue memory. Nevertheless, they are indications of the capacity of the body to learn from experience and store complex information at the cellular and tissue level.

Indications of the Release Process

The body's protective holding reaches muscles, ligaments, fascia, and all forms of connective tissue. It may be experienced as pain, limitation of motion, or restricted organ function. Both constriction and release occur at many levels. Memories, images, and emotions are often connected with physiological holding. The limitation or discomfort that we feel in one specific area is part of a broader picture of the body's protective adaptation to trauma or stress.

As we work with the client, we learn to recognize signs of change in the tissue and in the pattern of flow or congestion manifested by the body. When we touch with respect and support, muscles and connective tissue release and rebalance accumulated energy. There are many signals that the body is engaged in an inner process of release. Among these signs are the following:

- softening of muscle or ligament;
- micromovement of soft tissue or bone;
- release of heat energy experienced as warmth;
- uncomfortable sensations in the therapist's hand such as burning, prickling, numbing, or electricity;
- change in the pattern of breathing: anything from a small change of frequency to a big yawn or sigh;

- sounds from the belly because of increased intestinal tone and motility;

- eye movement behind closed lids;

- rapid flickering of closed eyelids;

- a pulsation beneath the therapist's hand or fingers that may feel like the cardiac pulse, but that unlike the heart pulse rises, peaks, and dissipates—the *therapeutic pulse;*

- a wave of emotion;

- a wave of physical pain;

- a perceptual sensation that seems to belong to another time and place;

- involuntary twitching or jerking of the body;

- a deep silence on every perceptual level;

- a pause in the craniosacral rhythm.

All of the above are indications that something is happening or has happened inside. Muscles and connective tissue appear to experiment with letting go of hypertonicity, modifying and balancing the customary level of activation they share among themselves. In the body, nothing happens in isolation. Any change will have some far reaching, if mild, effect on other parts. Therefore, the broader process of release involves not one muscle, joint, or ligament, but interacting networks of tissue, memories, and emotions.

Therapist and client may each experience different aspects of the release process. For instance, the client may feel a loosening and softening, while the therapist feels a brief pain in the hand or notices the client has released a sigh. After a release the tissue feels more at ease and alive.

We experience the release process as a waveform. That is, we feel a building of some indications, the signal reaches a peak, and then the sensation diminishes. This differentiates release from an intensification of symptoms. If some sense of heat, intense energy, pain, or emotion increases to a peak and persists, then my touch has triggered an intensification of symptoms, not release. In such a case I move gently away. My movement is not sudden, and it is usually small. I am looking for a position that gives support and enhances flow without triggering the symptom.

Responding to a Release

Are there specific things a therapist should do or say when a release occurs? This is a crucial question. It is important to realize that usually we do not need to make a change in what we do or say as we notice a release. Rather, we continue quietly in place. We maintain our touch and an attitude of respect, awareness, and support.

Awareness means that complementary awareness of self and client that we renew at every turn. Listen, notice, and attend to all the client manifests. In addition, listen, notice, and attend to all that rises up in you at this moment. Be especially aware of discomfort, physical or emotional, of memories or fears based on your own experiences. Be aware of any impulse to rush in and make things better for your client. On the other hand, if the process becomes intense, note the complementary desire to terminate the session as soon as possible.

Rather than sharing your personal insights and experience or escaping, this is the time to clear and center yourself. Remain calmly attentive, moving with the client but not attempting to influence the rate or direction of release. Simple phrases such as, "How are you doing?" or "Try to describe what is happening" may help the client acknowledge his or her experience by expressing it verbally. A quiet calmness in the therapist can be as powerful and reassuring as words.

At times therapists push for verbal revelations or ask leading questions based on their own experience. An emotional outpouring can be quite impressive and may secretly please the therapist. Yet, there is no evidence that such a release is more profound or beneficial than one signaled more quietly.

Rather, the most productive goal is to establish an environment of safety, security, and respect in which the client is free to explore the sources of his or her pain and restrictions and to release each at the appropriate time and place.

An inner shifting and balancing may continue for hours or days after a session. Changes are more solid and lasting when they occur as part of an organic process of rediscovery rather than as a reflection of contemporary society's desire to see quick results.

Is the client likely to get into some material that will be overwhelming to either client or practitioner? Experience has shown that when the therapist is attentive and respectful to both self and client, the client is ready for whatever release occurs. Trust that, without trying to influence it.

Appendix 2 offers additional thoughts on the verbal dialog between practitioner and client.

Why Start with the Body?

The introduction to this book describes the body's system of fascia, or connective tissue. The fascia extends in such a complex fashion throughout the body that a pattern of strain in any one area affects the balance in the whole system. We see such an adaptation when a person is suffering from a chronic knee or hip problem. As the body shifts and adjusts to the associated pain or misalignment, muscle and connective tissue find a new harmony. Posture changes in order to preserve functioning. Thus, the client frequently feels relief in the jaw or face as the pelvis releases. Conversely, a reduction of tension in the lower back will occur as the bones and fascia of the head release.

Because so much misalignment extends upward from the lower body and limbs to the upper back and neck, it is safer to start with the body and then move to the neck and head. Even when an injury has occurred primarily to the head, it is wise to check over and treat the body before addressing the head. Once the body is cleared, a more stable and properly functioning platform is ready to support the releases of the neck and head.

The Diaphragms

On the body, we will focus our efforts primarily on areas in which there is a large amount of connective tissue and muscle crossing the vertical axis. Because of the capacity of these areas to offer a flexible restraint on internal movement and flow, they have been collectively called *diaphragms*. The hyoid bone is not strictly a diaphragm. It is included here because of its importance for easing restrictions in the neck and throat.

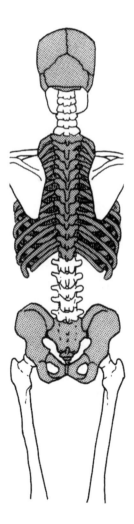

Figure 16. Skeletal Structure. The shading in this view helps to dramatize the change in skeletal form from wide structure to slender column. Craniosacral releases are utilized at each of these points of transition.

The release positions are

1. the pelvic floor, at the base of the torso;

2. the respiratory diaphragm, formed by the chief muscle of breathing;

3. the thoracic opening, where the neck meets the torso;

4. the hyoid bone in the throat; and

5. the cranial base, where the neck joins the head.

A dramatic change in skeletal structure and function naturally occurs at each of these locations. At both ends of the neck, a large and complex bony structure is attached to a slender column. Again, at both ends of the lumbar spine, in the lower back, a sturdy but single column of bones attaches to wide and complex bony structures. Obviously, these junctures are subject to unique forces.

The spine consists of three sections, based on function and structure: the slender column of bones forming the neck (cervical spine); the sturdier column of the chest (thoracic spine); and the bones of the more massive column in the lower back (lumbar spine).

Giving shape to the neck, and supporting the head, are seven cervical vertebrae, labeled C1 through C7 in descending order. In the chest (thorax), twelve thoracic vertebrae furnish a structural column for rib attachment and organ support. They are labeled T1 through T12. The lumbar spine is composed of five lumbar vertebrae, labeled L1 through L5. This last vertebra, L5, joins the sacrum.

The vertebrae of all sections are similar. An oval body, flattened at top and underneath, provides a weight-bearing surface, cushioned by a disc of cartilage. Behind the body is a bony structure forming an opening, like a ring, which provides a protective passageway for the spinal cord. The dura mater, the tough membrane lining the vault, forms a sleeve as it passes through the large opening (foramen magnum) in the occiput. This dural

Front

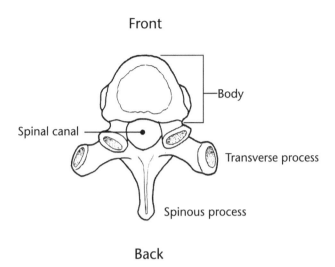

Spinal canal

Body

Transverse process

Spinous process

Back

Figure 17. A Typical Vertebra as Seen from Above. The oval body supports the weight of the entire column. The vertebral processes extending outward provide for both movement and stability by offering a surface for muscle attachment. The vertebrae are connected to each other by fibrous discs. Within these structures is a hollow space for the spinal canal.

---

sleeve extends through the canal created by these ringed openings, passing within the length of the spinal column and into the sacrum.

To the sides and to the rear of each vertebra are extensions, called *processes*. The transverse and spinous processes provide attachments for muscle and ligament, and establish range of motion between the vertebrae.

During these procedures, your client will lie face upward on a padded table. As therapist, use a chair or stool that you can easily move around the table. Your sensitivity and effectiveness are enhanced when you can sit comfortably with your legs extended under the table.

Have a pillow or other soft support available to place under the client's knees, as needed. A light blanket may be helpful, as certain clients become quite cool as they relax during a treatment.

1. The Pelvis

The pelvis forms a bowl, which contains and protects the organs of the lower torso: the digestive, eliminative, and sexual organs. The bowl itself is formed by the sacrum and the coccyx at the end of the spinal column, and the large, irregularly shaped hip bones on each side.

The hip bones curve around, providing leg sockets on each side, and joining in front at the pubic symphysis. This joint is given flexibility by a pad of cartilage, which buffers the meeting of the pubic bones at the center in the lower front.

On each side of the sacrum is a large, irregular surface, or facet, which meets the hip bone at the sacroiliac joint. The entire weight of the spinal column and upper body is transmitted to the hips and legs through these joints. A dense network of ligaments tightly binds together the sacrum and ilia.

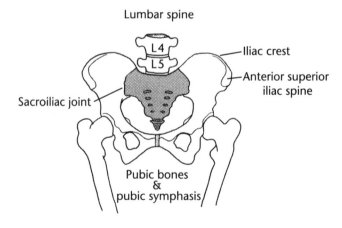

Figure 18. The Bones of the Pelvis. Attaching to the sacrum, which is shaded, the hip bones (ilia) spread outward and curve forward to form a bowl. The upper surface of the sacrum supports the lowest vertebra of the lumbar spine. The legs hinge at sockets on each side. (See also figure 24a.)

It is simple to palpate these features on yourself. Bring your hands to your waist on each side and slide them down so they rest on the curved upper edge of the hip bones. This upper surface is the iliac crest. Sliding forward along the crest, you can feel a point, the most forward (anterior) part of the hips. It is called the anterior superior iliac spine (ASIS). Sliding your fingers further downward and inward (toward the center) find the upper edge of the pubic bone crossing the lowest part of your abdomen. Gently investigate the width of this bone on yourself, on each side of the genital area.

Return your hands to your waist and the iliac crest. Now follow the crest around back, where it meets the bones and musculature of the lumbar spine. Directly down the center of the back, you can feel the rounded knobs of the spinous processes extending back from each vertebra. Where you seem to lose the iliac crest, feel directly downward on each side. Note the irregular vertical line of the sacroiliac joint where each hip bone meets the sacrum. Now place the heel of one hand directly between these joints. With fingers pointing downward, your hand can explore and get a sense of the shape of the sacrum, an inverted triangle terminating in the coccyx.

At the top of the sacrum is a large surface that joins the lowest bone of the lumbar spine: the fifth lumbar vertebra. Lying on your side to relax the muscles, again palpate the iliac crest, following to the back. Note that there is a space between the end of the iliac crest (posterior superior iliac spine) and the lumbar spine (backbone). The hips rise to each side above the juncture of sacrum and lumbar spine. Locate the sacrum again, between the sacroiliac joints. Notice the difference in feel between the flatter, cohesive surface of the sacrum and the rounded points of the spinous processes of the lumbar vertebrae. Flex your lower body and feel the movement of the spinous processes relative to one another and to the sacrum.

The spinal cord passes downward through a canal in the spinal column, distributing nerve fibers to the organs of the body through openings at every vertebra. The last nerve fibers continue through the canal at the fifth lumbar vertebra and are distributed to the body through openings in the sacrum.

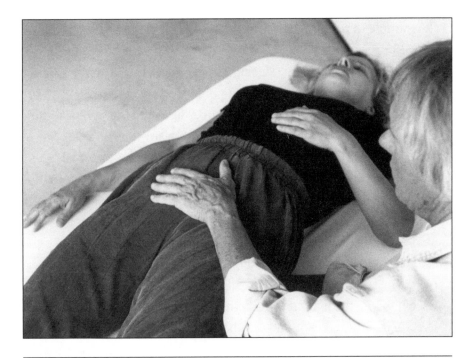

Figure 19. Releasing the Pelvic Diaphragm. Fingers of one hand contact the sacrum; the other hand rests on the lower abdomen at the edge of the pubic bone.

The sacrum itself begins life as a series of five bones, separated by discs. During the third decade of life, in the early or mid twenties, these bones fuse to form a rigid unit.

The joints of the sacrum are complex and unusual. The lumbosacral joint supports most of the weight of the spine and body above it. Thus it is the largest of the spinal articulations, and vulnerable to excessive pressure and sideways movement.

Joined to the end of the sacrum is the coccyx, a sort of mini-sacrum, composed of three or more fused segments of small size. It is an important attachment point for the muscles and ligaments of the pelvic floor.

The lower and outer edges of all these bony structures are important points of attachment for the muscles and ligaments forming the pelvic diaphragm. This forms a flexible floor for the entire torso.

The Pelvic Diaphragm

If the torso were simply closed at its base, like a section of rubber balloon, sources of stress would be greatly simplified. However, the pelvic diaphragm is structured to provide openings and organs for elimination, sexual intercourse, and childbirth. Within our societal context, these structures and functions become associated with hope, fear, pleasure, pain, and shame. Because of the strength of the emotional experiences focusing in this area, the fascia holds energies that influence functioning, alignment, and energy flow throughout the pelvis.

Our purpose here is to release unnecessary tensions stored in the soft tissues connecting and containing these structures and organs. This will release undue pressures on the bony structures, allowing freer range of movement and adjustment among themselves.

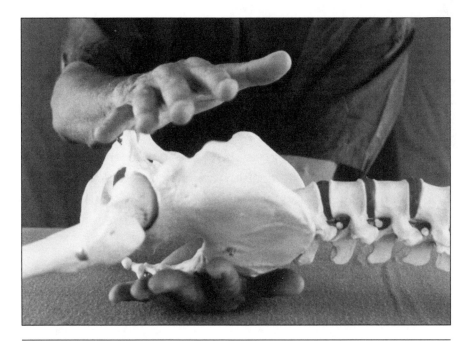

Figure 20. Releasing the Pelvic Diaphragm: A Skeletal View. We are facing the left hip. The therapist's left hand is at the sacrum, partially obscured by the hip bones. The right hand is spread over the lower abdomen, between the hip bones, just touching the pubic bone.

The pelvis, with its focus of physical pressures from the legs and body, and its focus of social and emotional pressures, is given to complex patterns of holding and pain. Despite this, our job is simple: provide a non-intrusive, supportive energy, facilitating any release that is appropriate for the moment.

Sit next to your client near the hips. With your client's assistance, coming directly from the side, place the hand that is nearer the client's head behind her hip so the fingers touch her sacrum. You may first want to find the sacrum on yourself and on your client in a standing position. Feel how your hand can conform to the bones and flesh so that it is most comfortable to you and your client.

Place your other hand, the hand nearer the client's feet, on the client's lower abdomen. Gently move it downward until the edge of your palm rests against the client's pubic bone. Apply a gentle and even touch, much as you did in the listening stations.

Let your arms and shoulders relax. Breathe easily. Maintaining a broad awareness, tune in to your client, and to yourself. Be aware of what you sense between your hands, as well as in your own arms and body.

You may perceive areas of tightness, relaxation, warmth, fluidity, hardness. You may perceive any of the indications of a tissue release with either hand.

In your first practices with this, there is no need to try to accomplish anything. Remain open and inquisitive: nurture an attitude of discovery. Stay for a few minutes, until you have perceived some sense of connection, movement, and therapeutic release. Then gently disengage your contact.

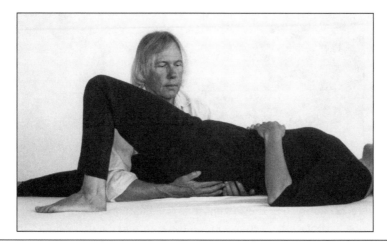

Figure 21. Releasing the Lumbosacral Joint. One hand contacts the sacrum, reaching from below. The fingers of the other hand stabilize the last lumbar vertebrae. Note: The client is pushing her foot against the table to lift the sacrum. She lowers her leg for the release.

The Lumbosacral Joint

Our purpose is to release any jamming or tightness between the sacrum and the lowest lumbar vertebrae, especially between S1 and L5. This is a very common source of discomfort and restricted motion in the lower back. Working in this area can give the client a tremendous sense of relief, and of lengthening.

As you sit facing your client's hips, your arm nearer the client's feet will rest on the table with the forearm extending upward so that your hand can contact the client's sacrum. There are two ways to accomplish this. The first, between the legs, requires longer arms and may be personally disturbing to some clients. Yet it provides the clearest sense of the sacrum and surrounding tissue. This is pictured in figure 21. The second, on a diagonal from the side, is much easier for the therapist, and may feel less intrusive to many clients.

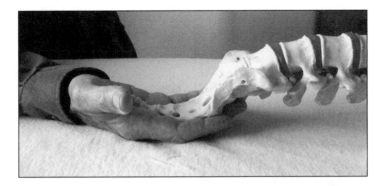

Figure 22. Contacting the Sacrum. This skeletal view shows the right hand in position to contact the sacrum and soft tissue around the pelvic floor. (The hip bones are not pictured.) Reaching the sacrum from below, the hand can sense the craniosacral rhythm more distinctly. The full hand does not cup the sacrum completely, because the heel of the hand would lift the pelvis and compress nearby tissue. Contact of the fingers lower on the sacrum is usually preferable.

In the first style, ask the client to bend the knee that is farther away from you and to push her foot on the table to lift the sacrum. As she does this, place your arm between the client's legs and contact the sacrum with the fingers of that hand. The client lowers her leg, and each person adjusts as necessary for comfort.

In the second style, support the client's knees with a cushion. This raises the upper legs so that you can slide your arm under the near leg to reach the client's sacrum in almost the same manner as above. The client may assist by rolling her hips slightly away from you as you place your hand. Adjust for the greatest comfort and sense of contact for each of you.

In either position, ensure that your hand and arm are comfortable. At times, the weight or bony structure of the sacrum is quite uncomfortable on the hand. Move your hand downward or spread your fingers to find an easier position. You can now feel the motion and the quality of the sacrum and surrounding tissue.

Try each of these styles so that you know how each feels and works for you. When you are comfortable in either style, it is time to place your other hand.

Our goal is to contact the lower lumbar vertebrae, in particular the fourth and fifth. With your free hand, feel the client's hip at the side and notice how high the hip bone extends. The top of the sacrum is a little below that level at the center of the back. Using the top of the hip as a guide, slide your free hand under the client's back until your fingertips can feel the points of the spinous processes, that is, the posterior extensions of the spinal vertebrae.

As you contact the client's sacrum, remember your palpation of this area on yourself. With your fingers, note the flat surface of the sacrum between the irregular lines of the sacroiliac joints and the transition above to spinous process with flat muscle on each side.

When you have a sense of where the last lumbar vertebra, L5, meets the upper segment of the sacrum, S1, then touch and maintain contact with the lower lumbar vertebrae. Make a clear, conscious contact with the points of the spinous processes through the intervening tissue. Usually the contact itself is sufficient for the following procedure.

Note the craniosacral rhythm of the sacrum, as it moves downward, tilts inward at the tip (coccyx), and returns. Consciously enhance this

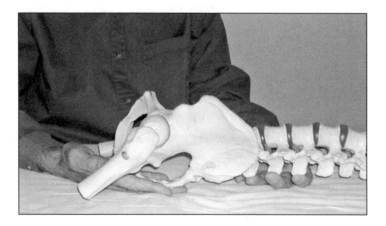

Figure 23. Releasing the Lumbosacral Joint: A Skeletal View. The right hand contacts the sacrum, sensing the craniosacral rhythm, while the fingers of the left hand stabilize the third, fourth, and fifth lumbar vertebrae. Note: Right and left are reversed when the therapist is sitting on the client's right.

movement, especially the downward component. This is as much by intention as by willed pressure. As your hand becomes attuned to the rhythm of the sacrum, merely think of assisting the downward component. Notice what is happening between your hand and the sacrum.

When you feel at ease with the subtle guidance of this movement, observe the sensations around the L5/S1 juncture. Does L5 move in total accord with the sacrum, or is there a sense of flexibility between the two? Our goal is flexibility.

Maintaining your conscious awareness of the rhythm, think of your hand as stabilizing the lumbar spine. That may mean a slight increase of pressure or a greater sense of contact. (Any force is very light.) Stay with this for a few cycles of the craniosacral rhythm as your other hand follows and enhances the motion of the sacrum. Then rest in place and merely observe.

You may notice any of the signs of a therapeutic release described in chapter 2. The craniosacral rhythm may stop for a while as the process of release occurs. Soft tissue and joints may discover a new balance. Merely stay in position during this process or until the rhythm returns.

At times, you may perceive some release or pulsation of energy, but when the rhythm returns the lumbar spine appears as tightly bound to the sacrum as before. Let it be for now. You have made a beginning. The next procedure may help to release this overly restricted bond.

The Sacroiliac Joints

A network of very dense fibrous connective tissue crosses the sacroiliac joint to attach the hip bone to the sacrum. In addition, there are strong muscles connecting the hip bone to the lower (lumbar) vertebrae. When there is considerable rigidity in the lower back, this entire complex of muscle and ligament holds these joints tightly together. Our purpose is to restore flexibility and range of motion among this group of joints and connections.

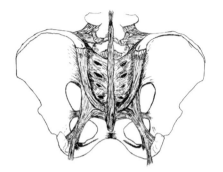

Figure 24a. Ligament Binding of the Pelvis. A view from behind, this drawing depicts the dense network of ligaments that secure the ilium to the sacrum on each side. Continuous bands of connective tissue reach upward along the spinal column and down to the "sit bones."

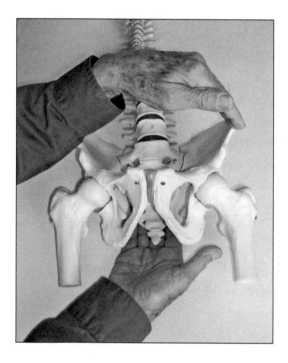

Figure 24b. Releasing the Sacroiliac Joints. A view from below, looking upward across the pubic bone to the sacrum and the lumbar spine (S1/L5). One hand contacts the sacrum from below, as shown in the two preceding photographs. The other arm bridges the anterior points of the hip bones. In the traditional release, this arm applies a light inward urge from each side, assisting the joints to release where the bones curve back to join the sacrum. (See also figure 18.)

Sitting beside the client, you may keep one hand where it has been, touching the sacrum from below. With your other hand, find the anterior points of the hip bones, the ASIS (anterior superior iliac spine). Place the fingers of that hand across the further point and contact the nearer point with your forearm. As you establish contact on each side, using your forearm and fingers, arch your arm over the belly. Are you comfortable? Shift your position if it helps you.

Notice the craniosacral rhythm, as the forward points of the hips expand outward and return. The traditional release is as follows. Working in harmony with the craniosacral rhythm, or any other energy you notice, gently bring the points of the hips (the ASIS) toward one another. The effect of this motion is to rotate the hip bones around a central axis so the sacroiliac joints at the client's back are expanded and released.

As you apply your presence and energy, go with the movement you sense, even if at first it is in the opposite direction than described here. Be aware of any sign of a therapeutic release around the sacrum. The effect of this procedure can be to ease restrictions in a wide area around the sacrum, including the juncture of the lumbar spine and sacrum.

I often find it simpler to assist in the release of each side separately. With one hand behind the sacrum, I bring my other hand to the hip on one side, conforming to the contour of the body. There I observe and follow the indications of a release process. When that side becomes quiet but freer, I move my hand to the other hip and repeat the process.

When the motion of the hips feels easier and freer, your job is done. Gently disengage and prepare to shift your position upward on the client's torso.

2. The Solar Plexus

Moving upward from the pelvic area, the upper end of the lumbar spine (L1) attaches to the twelfth and lowest of the thoracic vertebrae (T12). The twelve rib bones join and extend from each of the twelve thoracic vertebrae, meeting at the center of the chest to form a structure that provides stability, protection, and flexibility around the organs of the upper torso.

The tough, elastic sheet of muscle forming the respiratory diaphragm provides a physical separation between upper and lower torso. Immediately above are the lobes of the lungs. Below are the stomach, the spleen, the liver, the kidneys, the transverse large intestine, and the solar plexus, a large network of nerves supplying the abdominal organs. The windpipe and the esophagus, as well as numerous branches of the circulatory and nervous systems, pass through special openings in the diaphragm.

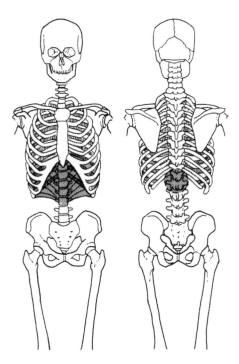

Figure 25. The Respiratory Diaphragm and the Solar Plexus. Shading on the front view illustrates the respiratory diaphragm attachments to the lower ribs and the upper lumbar vertebrae. Hand placement is near the center of the shaded area, with fingers overlapping the lower ribs. Shading on the back view circles the thoracic-lumbar juncture (T12/L1), the point supported by the practitioner's hand behind the client's body.

The respiratory diaphragm attaches to the lowest ribs and bubbles upward when at rest. During inhalation the muscle contracts or tightens, pulling downward. Pressure is reduced within the chest cavity and lungs, causing air to enter the lungs from the atmosphere. Simultaneously, diaphragm contraction presses downward on the contents of the lower torso, increasing internal pressure. The belly swells outward. At each inhalation internal pressure assists in the upward return of venous blood and lymph.

The area around the respiratory diaphragm hosts many important bodily functions and is a crossroads of physical energy. It is an area to which human experience has attributed many qualities: strength and vulnerability, courage and cowardice. Even our language reflects this: we speak of having guts or no guts; being hit in the guts; taking a breath before the plunge.

Fear and anxiety are often felt in the upper abdomen as a twisting of the stomach, a tightness of breath. Socially, we are urged to hold in our belly and stick out the chest, even at the expense of relaxed breathing. Experience of fear and anxiety, especially in a social context, can contribute to a visceral holding. This may be experienced as recurrent stomach pain, difficulty breathing, or a tendency to hold the breath when under stress.

Restriction of fascia and organ function around the respiratory diaphragm imposes added stress on the joint at T12/L1, where the broad bony structure of the chest meets the open abdomen, supported by the single column of lumbar vertebrae.

To palpate this region on yourself, start with your hands on your lower ribs, fingers almost meeting in front. Investigate the lower margin of the ribs, and the transition to your upper belly. Gently probe into the soft area beneath your ribs. How deep can you comfortably penetrate? Curl your fingers and carefully palpate under the lower edge of the ribs. With your fingertips you can sense the denser mass of the liver on the right side.

Investigate further the difference in feel between rib structure and abdomen. Notice this sensation of pressure directly in the middle under the ribs, where the solar plexus is located.

Now slide your hands around to the side and back, tracing the lower margin of the ribs to the spine. Palpate your own spine by feeling the points of the spinous processes. Notice changes of alignment and comfort across the transition from thoracic spine to lumbar spine. This is the area you support with one hand in the following procedure.

Our purpose is to aid in the release of restrictions that limit flow and full range of function throughout this area. The focus is especially on the T12/L1 juncture, relieving excessive pressure, restoring a more functional alignment.

Sit opposite the client's upper abdomen with your legs under the table. Place your hand that is nearer the client's head under his or her back so that it spans the T12/L1 juncture. Shift it so that both of you are satisfied with its position.

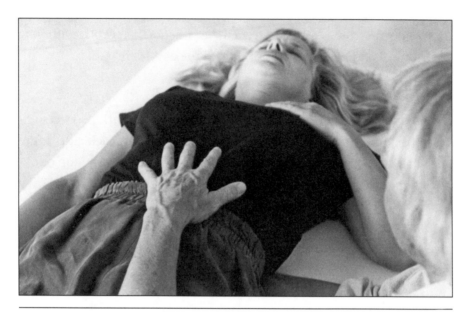

Figure 26. Releasing the Respiratory Diaphragm. One hand contacts the spine at the lower end of the rib structure (T12/L1). The other hand rests on the upper abdomen, tips of thumb and fingers extending over the lower ribs.

Place your other hand over the client's upper abdomen with fingers spread. The tips of your thumb and fingers will extend over the lowest ribs, while most of your hand will be resting on the belly below the ribs. As you establish contact through your hand, you may rest your forearm lightly on the client's lower body. Then bring your energy back to your center.

Attend to the subtle movements and sensations that you experience in your hands. You may sense your hands moving sideways, shifting in opposite directions, or rotating. This is part of the process of *unwinding,* that is, releasing a pattern of restrictions in the body tissues. Stay with this movement, adding your own presence and energy. Yet, there is no need to focus narrowly, or to impose a certain direction or sequence on the movement. The most will be accomplished by your awareness and presence as the body experiments with unraveling the imprint of restrictions from the past. Eventually you will feel a softening of the muscles of the back, or other indications of a therapeutic release. After that has occurred, you may want to stay in position for a few moments longer, enjoying the new sense of openness and calm that seem to be present. Then gently withdraw your contact and move your chair toward the end of the table.

3. The Thoracic Opening

In the upper torso, the shoulder girdle draws our attention. Two slender bones, the left and right clavicle, give definition on each side to the line where chest becomes shoulder. The clavicles attach at the top of the breastbone, below the throat, and extend laterally to each shoulder. They serve as the only bony attachment to the skeleton for the shoulder blades, shoulders, and arms. The entire structure of shoulder girdle and arms is invested with an amazing array of joints, muscles, nerves, and vessels establishing a functional harmony with the body.

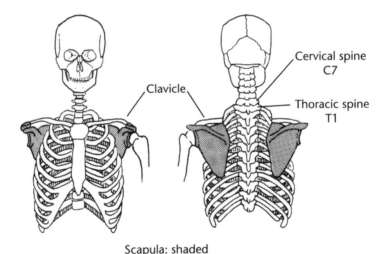

Scapula: shaded

Figure 27. The Thoracic Opening. The slender column of seven cervical vertebrae joins the broader and more massive structure of the thorax (chest). The shaded shoulder blades, the scapulas, which provide sockets for the arms, are attached to the larger skeleton by the clavicle bones. For the release, one hand is placed behind, supporting the C7/T1 juncture. The other hand rests on the upper chest, using the clavicles as reference points.

Intimately involved with this fascinating complex, rising above its base on the first thoracic vertebra, T1, is the slender column of seven cervical vertebrae forming the neck. Muscles providing movement and stability for the neck and the head meet and blend with muscles providing lift and movement for the shoulders and the upper arms. These muscles extend from cervical vertebrae to shoulder blades and upper ribs, from clavicles to neck and base of skull, from spine and ribs to shoulder blades and upper arms.

In the human structure, the vast amounts of musculature attaching to the neck, the head, the shoulders, and the ribs provide versatility of movement as well as protection. Yet, the size and weight of the head, the number of vertebrae on which it is supported, and the types of kinetic forces that an active person experiences tend to make this a vulnerable area. The amount of muscle and fascia engaging in such a variety of functions means that when trauma is imprinted within the tissues, there is a wide range of possibilities. This is seen in therapeutic practice when restrictions in the shoulder and upper chest have an influence extending to the neck, the jaw, and the face.

We are working with the roof of the torso, in particular the roof of the rib-enclosed thorax, and its opening via the neck to the head. This region might be compared to the main trunk line of a communications system as it leads from (or toward) the communication center. For proper functioning, lines of communication and power and resources for nourishment and repair must be open and flowing in each direction.

For the individual, this is a crucial pathway for personal expression. The voice emerges from the chest and throat. We express facets of our identity, personality, love, and work through facial expressions and with the actions of our shoulders, arms, and hands.

Therapeutic experience suggests that the more crucial component of expression for an individual flows not from the rational mind but from the heart and body. Aiding in clearing the "pathways of expression" for an individual often entails repeated attention to the heart and the shoulders as well as the throat and the base of the neck.

The impact of traumatic emotional experience can lead to restrictions in the upper chest and shoulders that influence freedom of verbal expression and freedom of physical movement in the shoulders, neck, face, and voice.

To palpate this region on yourself, first explore with one hand the contour of your upper chest. Note the curved lines of ribs meeting sternum on each side, and the hollow or softness between ribs. Move upward and follow the clavicle on each side until it meets the shoulder. Holding the clavicle, move that shoulder forward and back, up and down. Notice how far clavicle and shoulder can lift from the torso as defined by the ribs.

Reach behind your back, and find the inner edge of your opposite scapula (shoulder blade). Notice how the scapula slides over the back, across the ribs, as you raise your shoulder or rotate it forward.

Finally, place the palm of your hand on your upper chest. Spread your fingers so that the thumb rests on the clavicle on the near side, the index and middle fingers on the clavicle on the other side. Feel the contour beneath your hand, and sense the energy between hand and chest. This is a hand position you will use in the following procedure.

Sit almost at the upper corner of the treatment table, at the client's neck and shoulder. Bring one hand diagonally toward the base of the neck, placing it under the back and neck so the palm bridges the C7/T1 juncture. You may feel the spinous processes, the muscle on each side of the spine, and perhaps the edge of the shoulder blades. Position your fingers so they are comfortable.

Place your other hand on the client's upper chest. Spread your thumb away from your fingers so that you can rest your thumb and index finger on the clavicles extending to each side.

Bring your awareness to the fingers and palms of both hands. You may find that you can work with less strain if you let your forearm rest lightly on the client's chest. Consult with your client and experiment with this.

Follow the direction of unwinding or release, moving with the tissue, varying pressure and position when you feel drawn to do so.

If you have time, and feel drawn to it, let your hands move to one or the other of the shoulders, where you may also experience unwinding and

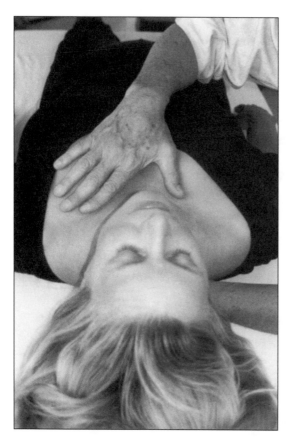

Figure 28. Releasing the Thoracic Opening. One hand is behind, comfortably supporting the spine at the neck and upper back. Notice the arm is on a diagonal between the neck and shoulders. It does not lift the shoulders. The other hand rests on the chest, index finger and thumb spread to contact the clavicles. If this arm can rest on the client's body, then the practitioner's shoulder is able to relax.

therapeutic release. There are many areas of potential constriction in the upper torso, the release of which contributes to the freedom of movement and flow at the thoracic inlet and above.

4. The Hyoid Bone

There is one bone in the human body that does not directly join with other bones in the skeletal frame. It is the hyoid bone. Roughly semicircular in shape, it floats between the base of the tongue and the thyroid cartilage at the front of the throat. It is anchored below by muscle and membrane to the thyroid cartilage and to the sternum. To the sides and above it anchors cartilage and musculature, which form the floor of the mouth, and function in chewing, swallowing, and speech.

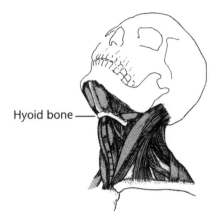

Hyoid bone ——

Figure 29. The Hyoid Bone. The hyoid is a semicircular bone in the throat, beneath the tongue and above the thick cartilage at the top of the windpipe. It is an important point of attachment for muscles involved in chewing, swallowing, and speech. Fingers gently contact the bone from each side for the hyoid release.

To palpate the hyoid bone on yourself, bring one hand to your throat, thumb on one side, fingers on the other. With thumb and index finger trace the cartilage of your trachea (windpipe) from the base of your neck to the prominent thyroid cartilage (the Adam's apple). Feel the upper edge of this cartilage. Moving your fingers just above this edge, let them sink into the soft tissue until you are aware of a bony surface. This is the hyoid bone. When you swallow, both the hyoid and the thyroid cartilage will move up and down. When you speak, the thyroid cartilage vibrates and the hyoid moves.

If you let your fingers sink directly back into the musculature of the neck, you can find a pulse. This is the region of the carotid artery and jugular vein. It is important to keep clear of these to assure normal blood flow to the brain.

Because the mouth and face are so important in expressiveness, communication, and obtaining nourishment, the mouth and the associated structures of the lower face and neck are vulnerable to imprints of trauma and pain as well as love and nurturing.

Our purpose is to release imprints of trauma and restriction in the muscles and fascia attached to the hyoid bone in the throat. This is a beginning in opening the channels through which we share expressiveness and nurturing. Looking at it physiologically, we are aiding in the release of the muscles and connective tissues of the throat. The next section of this chapter deals with the muscles and fascia at the back of the neck.

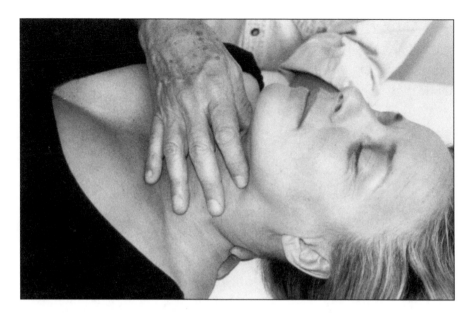

Figure 30. Releasing the Hyoid. One hand makes contact behind the neck. The thumb and index finger of the other hand lightly grasp the hyoid bone, above the projecting cartilage of the larynx (the Adam's apple).

Sitting at an upper corner of the treatment table as in the previous release, place your hand that is closer to the client's head under his or her neck. From the hand position of the thoracic inlet release, you may now slide your hand upward so that it covers the back of the neck. Then rest the edge of the other hand lightly on the breastbone, near the clavicles. This provides a stable platform as you touch the throat.

With your thumb and forefinger, lightly contact the sides of the client's windpipe. Slide upward, slightly above the most prominent cartilage of the windpipe, the Adam's apple, to where the neck flares outward to merge into the chin and lower jaw. Allow your thumb and forefinger to sink into the tissue as you establish contact. The notion of letting your fingers sink into the tissue, rather than pushing in, is important. If you wait a few moments, the tissue will let your fingers in, and you will be more successful in the procedure.

If you feel the cardiac pulse, shift your contact away from the pulse, staying just above the upper edge of the windpipe. If your client speaks or swallows, you will be able to feel the hyoid bone and its connecting tissue moving or vibrating beneath your fingertips.

When you are satisfied that you are in contact with the hyoid, and your client is comfortable with your touch, center yourself and tune in to the movement and energy between your fingers. Follow and enhance this movement, using light pressure.

Be aware of your own sensations. How is it for you to have someone touch your throat? How do you feel having such a grasp of another person's throat? Are you breathing easily? Are your shoulders relaxed? What have you noticed of your client's breathing and muscle tension?

Tune in to the signs of therapeutic release, including heat release into your hand behind the client's neck. This release can be a helpful preparation for releasing the tensions at the back of the neck and for later work on the client's head.

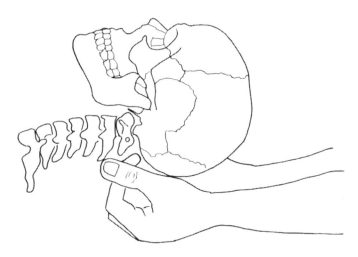

Figure 31. The Atlanto-occipital Release: A Skeletal View. The occiput is supported by the heel of each hand, creating space for the fingers to palpate the junction of neck and occiput. Fingertips slide along the occiput as neck muscle and fascia soften.

5. The Base of the Skull: The Atlanto-occipital Joint

The entire spine is laced with muscles that link each vertebra to the next one, two or three above and below. Other muscles cross from spinous process at the middle to attachments on the transverse processes at the sides of vertebrae above and below. These muscles provide stability and facilitate bending and twisting movements along the spine and neck. More massive muscle groups run most of the length of the spine, on each side. They provide movement, strength, and support. All of these muscle groups continue at the back of the neck and attach in some manner to the base of the skull. In addition, muscles extend from the cervical vertebrae and the base of the skull to the upper ribs and the shoulders.

The occiput, or base of the skull, is positioned at the top of the cervical column by means of facets, smooth joint surfaces on the bone. The joint is aligned so that the foramen magnum, the large opening in the skull base, is directly above the spinal canal. The musculature described ensures that the skull is firmly positioned at the top of the spine, yet has ample provision for a complex set of movements.

When any of these muscles and fascia is chronically tight, vertebrae may be pulled out of alignment, causing pain and restricted motion of the head and neck. A particular example of misalignment occurs between the occiput and C1. The occiput becomes jammed against the first verte-bra, and pulled forward at its base, encroaching upon and stressing the dural tube.

To palpate this area on yourself, place the fingers of one hand along the points of the spinous processes at the back of the neck. Feel the movement in the vertebrae as you move your head right and left, up and down.

Next, holding your neck with one or both hands, feel the action of the muscles at side and back as you again move your head in every direction.

Finally, bring the fingers of both hands to the back of the skull. Begin with index fingers on each side of the protuberance directly in back. Slide your fingers down, feeling the contour of the occiput. Notice the thickening and softening that occurs with muscle attachment at the lower back of the occiput. Search through the muscle to find the skull as it curves to

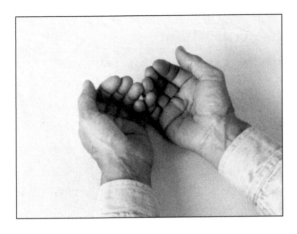

Figure 32. The Atlanto-occipital Release: Finger Positions. The fingers of each hand curl back so fingertips contact the occiput.

meet the cervical spine. The widening you feel just behind the ears is the mastoid process of the temporal bone. The temporal bones, the parietal (side) bones, and the occiput join at sutures in this area. In releasing the cranial base, your fingers will slide along the base of the occiput into the muscle immediately at the back of the neck.

Our purpose is to aid in easing muscles and fascia in this area, making it possible for the base of the skull to float more freely above the cervical vertebrae. In the process, there is often considerable release of constriction in the tissue at the back of the neck, experienced by the clinician as heat or pulsation, and by the client as deep relaxation of the neck.

Move your chair to the head of the treatment table. Sit so your feet and knees are comfortably under the table and you can rest you forearms on the table. You may need to ask your client to move down the table so that you can place your hands under his or her head and gain support for your forearms. Usually you will be more comfortable if your chair is a little lower than it has been for the preceding releases on the body.

Place your hands palm upward beside the client's head. Slide both hands under the occiput, the back of the head, so that you can cradle the head comfortably. Lift the client's head with the heels of your hands. This gives space behind the neck. Now begin to feel with your fingers, discovering how the muscles of the neck attach to the base of the skull.

With the three middle fingers on each hand, find the sensitive line where neck muscles reach downward from the skull. Gently lower the cli-

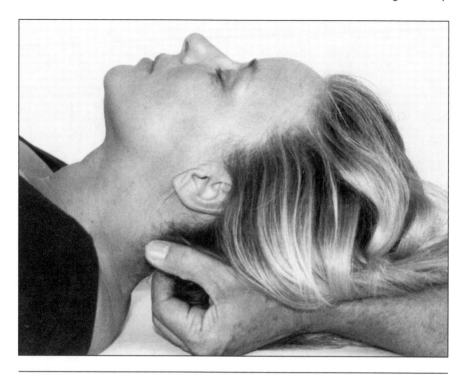

Figure 33. Hands in Place for the Atlanto-occipital Release. The middle two
or three fingers of each hand slide along the base of the skull, sinking into
the softening neck muscle. As the muscle and fascia yield, the angle of the fingers
is adjusted, so the fingers continue in contact with the occiput as they penetrate
deeply into the soft tissue. The weight of the head is adjusted by continuing
to support the head on the heels of the hands.

ent's head with the heels of your hands, so that your fingers press against
the soft tissue at the base of the skull.

Reposition your hand and fingers as needed so that your fingertips
maintain contact with the occiput. Let your fingertips slip along the base
of the skull as the muscle and connective tissue soften.

You may notice a great difference in tightness from one side to the
other. The muscles may go through cycles of loosening and tightening. It
may be useful to describe these to your client and to state your purpose:
to assist the neck muscles to relax so that the joint above the neck may
experience greater freedom.

Often you will experience considerable heat and a sense of intensity in your fingertips. You may shift your position slightly, for comfort, and to maintain an effective angle with your fingers.

Important considerations: Your fingertips continue to maintain an angle so that they slip along the base of the skull as the neck muscle relaxes. As this release progresses, continue to support most of the weight of the head with the heels of your hands. The pressure exerted comes from the weight of the head, rather than from a thrusting of your fingers. You are patient, observant, and at one with this process, so that you can assist in it, rather than making it happen.

As the muscles soften and you feel your fingertips penetrating the tissue, visualize the two hands rotating outward, so that the tips of the fingers spread the muscle slightly away from the centerline. I say "visualize" so that you let this happen, or follow the tissue, rather than pushing it.

As you reach a sense of completion with this release, relax your fingers and slide your hands upward (toward you) so that you cradle the client's head. This is an opportunity to look (inwardly sense) along the entire spine.

Visualize the dural tube as it passes through the foramen magnum at the base of the skull and extends through the spinal canal of the neck and upper back.

Notice the component of the craniosacral rhythm that appears to pull downward on the occiput, then release it. With your intention and a light touch, enhance this rhythm. What do you perceive in the dural tube? Within the first few vertebrae? Further down the spine? Do you or your client notice a sense of lengthening in the spine? Remain with this for a few minutes, until you have a sense of completion or an eagerness to move on. Then gently release the head and disengage. You are ready to move to the cranial releases in the next chapter. Before continuing, notice how you feel in your arms and shoulders. Stretch and move if this helps to relax your muscles.

Chapter 3

The Cranial Releases

This chapter brings us to the final portion of a craniosacral session. The cranial releases are treated in a separate chapter because of their special nature. The quality of awareness and respect emphasized in the previous chapter is even more important here. The diaphragm releases deal with broad areas of body tissue and structure. The head is unique in the large number of releases within such a small area.

In the circumscribed realm of the head, we pay attention to very specific locations and interconnections. One after the other, we will assist in the release of a set of contiguous bones and connective tissue. As we work at one location, then another, we address the fascia, especially the dura mater, from one direction, then another.

Despite the confined and specific focus of our work with the head, there is tremendous interaction with the body. During the releases of the body, clients often note a return of ease in jaw and face. Even when the major problem or complaint is in the pelvis, connections turn up in the upper body and the head. Conversely, as we perform these specific releases around the cranial vault, clients often report sensations of energy change or easing in shoulders, chest, abdomen, and pelvis.

The cranial releases round off the work begun with the listening stations and diaphragm releases. The work of the body is not complete without attention to the head. Nor would adjustments within the cranial vault be complete without attention to the important bodily manifestations of constriction and imbalance.

By performing the work of this and the preceding chapter, both you and your client experience the reality of the organism as a whole, interconnected physical being. Moreover, each of you experiences from your own perspective the effectiveness of an integrated craniosacral treatment.

The following section reviews the anatomy of the head in preparation for the cranial releases. Part 2, chapter 7 contains a further description of cranial anatomy.

Anatomical Survey

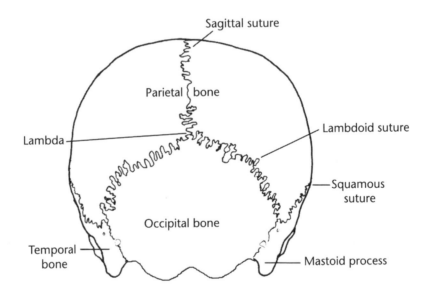

Figure 34. The Occiput and the Sutures at the Back of the Skull. The irregular, wandering path of the joint provides a secure yet living connection between the cranial bones. Here, the sagittal and lambdoid sutures meet at lambda, joining the parietal and occipital bones. A portion of the squamous suture is visible at each side where the temporal bones join the parietal bones.

The bony framework of the head, face, and neck is a masterpiece of integrated, functional construction. More than twenty bones are linked by a specialized joint, the suture. The suture provides a secure interlocking of edges, similar to that provided by interlacing the fingers. The soft connective tissue of the periosteum, enlivened with blood vessels and nerve endings, lines the sutures, providing for flexibility and give between parts. The entire structure is a flexing, responsive, interactive complex of substructures. It has the capacity to respond to differentials of inner and outer pressure and to adapt to impact and stress.

The large, curved bones of the cranial vault, lined with the dura mater and cushioned by cerebrospinal fluid, provide a protective and nurturing environment for the delicate mass of nerve tissue constituting the brain. The dura mater links the bones of the cranial vault to one another with a tough yet elastic membrane.

In effect, it is as if an elastic capsule had been formed and the cranial bones were set into its sticky outer surface. Thus the cranial bones interact with one another at their sutures, and they interact with the elastic capsule, the dura mater, in which they are embedded. The elastic quality of the connective tissue allows responsiveness to the environment.

On the other hand, the dura mater can limit responsiveness. As a connective tissue, or fascia, the dura mater can hold the imprint of past trauma and stress, which means it can be restricted in the range of its response, ready to react protectively and more rapidly if a similar traumatic circumstance arises.

Imagine again that all of the cranial bones are embedded in the dura mater, as if on the surface of a balloon. Imagine cold air causes the balloon to shrink. It pulls in on itself, pulling the bones toward one another, jamming them together along their edges.

This is one way to understand the interaction of cranial bones, sutures, and dura mater. A restriction at one location in the cranial vault will cause asymmetric movement of nearby structures. Other bones adapt to the limitations of energy and movement. Thus, a restriction of the dura mater can be amplified throughout the skull and into the spine.

It is the dura mater, in particular, that we address as we work with the bones of the cranial vault. Our therapeutic presence and touch help encourage movement and flexibility at the edges of bones, releasing restrictions in the dura mater that have fixed the bones together rigidly. The bones of the head and face are the points of contact through which we reach the dura mater, facilitating unwinding and therapeutic release.

Thus, our goal is to facilitate release of restrictions of movement and flow among the bones and fascia of the cranial vault. We will also address the lower jaw, or mandible. The mandible acts as a long lever, anchored into the temporal bones at the side of the head and moved by very strong muscles. Thus, the lower jaw exerts considerable leverage on the bones of the head.

The Pattern of Release

The pattern of release is often similar among these bones. Often, the first sensation experienced is not movement, but energy pulsing or shifting within the head. Sometimes the bone beneath the skin feels hard. This suggests constriction in the dura mater and in connective tissue that covers the bone and lines the sutures. The movement may appear as a tilting or twisting rather than a balanced and full rhythm. This motion is usually the result of localized constriction at the sutures hampering free movement of bones in that area.

Our touch evokes a response in the connective tissue and in the dura mater. We may connect with restriction and release in the immediate area and in the entire elastic capsule of the cranial vault. Constriction eases and returns as the tissue searches through a pattern of holding and release, searching for a freer and more harmonious level of holding. Therefore, we may feel movement, then hesitation, movement and hesitation. Immediate restriction eases; then restrictions that are more distant adjust to a new configuration of tightness and flexibility in the entire capsule.

The decision that the release of a particular region is complete is partly intuition, partly sensation, partly arbitrary. The bone seems to move with greater ease, more evenly and in a broader range: it maintains its connection with neighbors, yet has gained resilience. Bone that felt hard at first feels more alive later.

Even when some constriction remains, the release obtained may be adequate. There is something to be said for partially releasing each bone in sequence, gently easing the entire cranial vault to greater flexibility and responsiveness, rather than trying to get maximum release at a specific location.

We will address the bones in an order that is dictated partially by the nature of their interconnected structure. The bones in their order of approach are

1. the frontal bone, or forehead;

2. the parietal bones, the upper posterior sides of the skull;

3. the sphenoid, the inner floor of the cranial vault;

4. the temporal bones, the lower posterior sides of the skull;

5. the mandible, or lower jaw; and

6. the occiput and the still point.

The Quality of Touch: The Question of Pressure

We sometimes wonder how much pressure to use on the bones of the head. The question itself can be misleading. In recent years I have abandoned the use of the term *pressure*. The most effective intervention is comprised of presence and supportive touch.

Practitioners working from a concept of proper alignment will apply strong or sudden pressure to overcome resistance. Some of this approach has carried into craniosacral therapy. However, as craniosacral practice has developed the approach has changed. We have learned to attune ourselves to small movements of body structures, facilitating release through presence and support. As we gain experience, we usually find that the body is leading us very well. The key is to touch with sensitivity and broadened perception rather than with pressure.

Self-palpation

Before beginning to work on your client, it will be helpful to explore these bones on yourself.

Frontal Bone

Bring your hands up, as if covering your face. With fingers spread across your forehead, lightly contact the anterior surface of the frontal bone. Notice how the bone curves upward across the top and turns more sharply at each side, near your temples. You can feel the lower edge of the frontal bone at the base of your fingers.

Now lower your hands so that you can trace the lower edge of the frontal bone at your eyebrows, above the orbits of your eyes. Follow the edge of the bone to each side and investigate the soft temple area, just beyond the eyebrow. An extension of the sphenoid bone curves upward here, forming a suture with the frontal.

Returning your hands to the front of your face, again contact the anterior surface of the frontal bone. Now bring your fingers upward, past

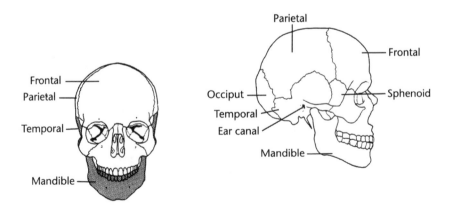

Figure 35. The Bones of the Head Addressed in the Cranial Releases.
You may also consult the illustrations in part 2, chapter 7.

your hairline. Search for the slight irregularity on the surface of the skull that marks the line of the coronal suture. The coronal suture is almost as deep into the hairline as the eyebrows are below the hairline. Along this suture, the frontal bone meets the two parietal bones.

You can also follow the coronal suture upward. Place two or three fingers over the soft temple at the end of each eyebrow. Describe a quarter circle up and back from the eyebrow, around this soft area. Then explore upward for the irregularity between frontal and parietal bones. The coronal suture extends from just behind and above the temple area, upward to bregma.

Bregma is the point on the centerline of the skull, along the coronal suture, where both parietal bones contact the frontal bone. In a newborn child, it is the center of a soft spot, or fontanel. Investigate the location of the coronal suture and bregma, and get a sense of the size and shape of the frontal bone.

Again, bring your hands and fingers to the starting position, covering the frontal bone. Let your fingers spread enough so your index fingers pass the rounded edge at each side to lightly grip the frontal bone. While the other fingers remain in contact with the forehead, explore the sensation of lifting anteriorly (to the front) with the side surface of the index fingers.

Breathe evenly and calmly. Remain with this until you experience that such a light touch does actually have an effect. Then gently release.

Parietal Bones

Bring your hands to the sides of your head, with two or three fingers on the soft temple. Beneath your fingers, below the soft tissue, is an extension of the sphenoid bone. Directly behind the temple, this rounded segment of the sphenoid joins the temporal bone. Now bring your fingers back, forming a semicircle just above and behind the ears. Your fingers enclose the temporal bone. Explore up and down, searching for the soft and sensitive line of the squamous suture joining the temporal and parietal bones. The suture begins just above and behind the soft temple, and forms a half circle, just above and then behind the ears. This suture tends to have a soft feel, and may be sensitive to touch.

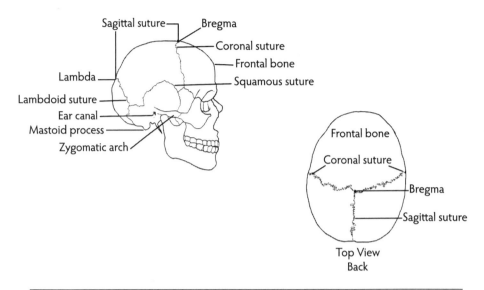

Figure 36. A Reference Guide to the Significant Features of the Cranium.
For the occiput, please refer to figure 34.

After exploring the squamous suture between the temporal and parietal bones, again locate the coronal suture, between the frontal and parietal bones. At the top centerline of the skull, beginning at the point bregma, the two parietal bones are joined in the sagittal suture. Resting your hands lightly on each side of your head, behind the coronal suture, your fingers will be on the parietal bones. Explore the sagittal suture with your fingers. From bregma, directly behind the frontal bone, follow the line of sensitivity back and down, to lambda.

Lambda is the point just above the very back of the head where the two parietal bones meet the occipital bone. The occipital protuberance lies below this point.

The suture between the parietal bones and the occiput extends down and to each side from lambda. This suture is called the lambdoid suture because when viewed from behind it is shaped like the Greek letter lambda: Λ.

Explore the lambdoid suture with your fingers, following the line of sensitivity down and outward from the point lambda. The suture continues down past the area where neck muscles attach to the base of the skull. However, the parietal bone curves away from the occiput just above the level of the ear canal, forming a corner where the temporal bone meets the occiput.

You have traced the major sutures of the parietal bone, describing its area on each side of your head. Trace the sutures again to confirm your sense of the size and shape of the two parietal bones.

Now bring your hands to the sides of your head, your fingertips along the sagittal suture, your palms contacting the parietal bones. Slide your fingertips down each side, rounding the sharp curve of the parietal bone, until you reach the squamous suture above the ears, at the temporal bone.

In working with the parietal bones, your fingertips will be above this sensitive suture, at the ridge on the side, just before the parietals curve around to form the upper surface of the skull. Explore this area: above the ears and the squamous suture; behind the frontal bone and the coronal suture. Holding your fingers still, can you sense movement, the craniosacral rhythm?

Apply a light touch inward. Note the sensation within your skull. Then imagine that the bones are moving upward, toward the space above your head. Note that sensation. These are motions traditionally used in releasing the parietal bones.

Occiput

When we cradle the client's head in our hands, the occiput rests in our palms. Our fingers extend beyond the inward curve of the occiput to the neck muscles. To explore this area on yourself, bring your fingers again to the lambdoid suture on each side of the external occipital protuberance. The upper part of the occiput is contained within this roughly triangular region. As you slide your fingertips downward along the suture, note that the bone swells outward on each side of the suture. Just behind the ear is the rounded mastoid process of the temporal bone. Toward the center from this, across the suture, the occiput also swells outward slightly. (See figure 34.) These swellings of temporal bone and occiput are regions of attachment for powerful neck muscles. In fact, these rounded sections of bone are developed after birth by the continual action of muscles holding and turning the head.

Feel the muscles attaching all across the base of the skull. These have an important effect on the quality of sutures and the rhythm throughout the cranium. When the neck is chronically tight, the cranial sutures respond by holding more firmly against that pull. Easing of neck muscles and occipital sutures is very helpful for comfort throughout the cranium and jaw.

The occiput curves inward between the temporal bones on each side. It meets the sphenoid at the sphenobasilar synchondrosis. The spinal column joins the head within this hidden section of the occiput, between the temporal bones.

Sphenoid Bone

Return your palms to the sides of your face, with one or two fingers on the soft temple. You will not feel bone directly beneath the skin. The surface of the skull is recessed to provide a channel for muscle fibers to the mandible (lower jaw). You can feel the action of this muscle when you clench and release your teeth.

It is through the soft tissue of the temple that we contact the sphenoid bone, part of the floor of the cranial vault. Here the sphenoid curves upward on each side to form wall as well as floor. These extensions are known as the greater wings of the sphenoid.

With your hands along the sides of your face and your fingers on the temples, attune yourself to the greater wings of the sphenoid, beneath the muscle fiber. With the craniosacral rhythm the sphenoid moves downward with each expansion of the cranial vault, then returns upward. Follow the rhythm for a few cycles; then release your contact.

Zygomatic Arch

Directly below the temples, you can feel the zygomatic arch forming a ridge from the zygoma (cheekbone), almost to the ear canal. The muscle covering the temple travels under this arch.

Temporal Bones

Now return to the temporal bone: with the fingertips of both hands, find the squamous suture slightly above your ears. Follow around and down behind your ears. Behind the lower half of the ear, the temporal bone curves to meet the occiput. The suture passes through a flattened area behind and below the ear canal. Close behind the ear is a rounded knob, the mastoid process. The mastoid process is a point of ligament and muscle attachment on the temporal bone, and a reference point in our work.

Rest your index finger on the mastoid process. Stabilize your middle finger by placing it directly in your ear canal, and place your fourth finger on the zygomatic arch, directly in front of the ear canal. In this position, it is possible to sense a rotation of the temporal bone with the cycle of the craniosacral rhythm. The components of the craniosacral rhythm on the temporal bone will be discussed more fully when the release is described.

Mandible

The mandible, with the teeth, gives shape to the lower jaw. It meets the temporal bone in an unusual joint, hinging downward and sliding forward as the mouth opens. Bringing your hands to the sides of your face, place your fingers along the ridge formed by the zygomatic arch, with your index fingers up against the cartilage flap anterior to the ear canal. Moving your jaw in different directions, explore the sensation of the mandible moving on its joint, the temporomandibular joint (TMJ).

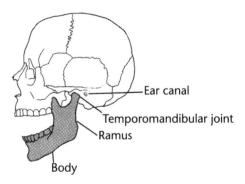

Ear canal

Temporomandibular joint

Ramus

Body

Figure 37. The Mandible. A side view, shaded. The temporomandibular joint hinges immediately in front of the ear canal.

Next, place the fingers of both hands along the sides of the jaw, so your little fingers are at the chin. This is the body of the mandible. With your fingers and thumb, explore the lower edge, finding the notch just before the bone turns upward, toward the ear. The section of the mandible that reaches upward on each side is known as the ramus. Feel its breadth beneath the muscle that cloaks it.

The ramus branches into two short sections. The posterior branch of the ramus hinges at the temporal bone just in front of the ear canal.

The anterior branch of the ramus slides beneath the zygomatic arch. By placing your fingers just below the zygomatic arch, you can feel that part of the mandible slide out and in as you open and close your mouth.

Now bring your hands lower, with your fingers along the line of your jaw. At the posterior corner of the jaw, your index finger will rest in thicker muscle. With the thumb of each hand, find the notch along the lower edge of the jaw, under the muscle pad.

Breathing quietly, notice sensations of energy and movement in the mandible and its joint.

The Cranial Releases

You have completed your introductory exploration of the bones and joints of the head and face. We now turn to the actual cranial releases.

The Frontal Bone

As part of the cranial vault, the frontal bone is embedded in, or lined with, the tough membrane of the dura mater. With the ethmoid bone, it serves as the anterior attachment for the falx cerebri, a sheet of membrane partially separating the two sides of the brain. A fold of the dura mater, this tough, stabilizing membrane stretches front to back in the cranial vault, attaching to the frontal bone and occiput and to the parietal bones along the sagittal suture.

The traditional first step in releasing restrictions in the movement of cranial bones is to lift the frontal bone forward from the cranial bones with which it articulates, in particular the parietal and sphenoid bones.

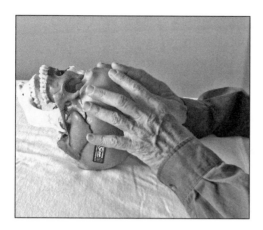

Figure 38a. Finger Positions
on the Frontal Bone.

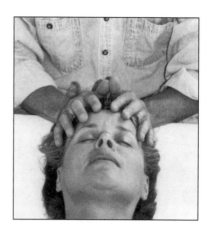

Figure 38b. Hands in Place
for the Frontal Release.

The table supports the therapist's arms. The fingers are spread as they lightly touch the forehead. The palms and thumbs are not touching the head.

Through the frontal bone, we address restrictions in the dura mater and in the falx cerebri.

Your client is lying face up on the treatment table. By this time in the session, a pillow or bolster under the knees may be helpful for comfort and will help relieve the lower back. The client's hands and arms are comfortably positioned at the sides, or resting on the body.

Sit at the head of the table, with your legs and knees under the table. Ensure that you have enough space to rest your forearms on the table as you contact your client's head. An extension for the table helps, or your client can move a few inches toward the foot.

To begin, rest your forearms or elbows on the table. Then, bring your hands to your client's head, placing four fingers of each hand on the forehead. Sliding sideways, explore the curve on each side of the frontal bone. On the side, just beyond the curve, there is often a slight ridge. Place the ring finger of each hand on each side at this ridge. The other fingers rest lightly on the forehead.

In some clients, the frontal bone is more evenly rounded, and the ridge is not obvious. In this case, rotate your hands by moving your wrists outward and angle several fingers across the curve from each side. Use this increased finger surface to contact the frontal bones from each side.

Your thumbs will touch each other or cross, not contacting the head. Your other fingers on the forehead provide a presence and a stabilizing influence, which is beneficial to this release.

Having carefully placed your hands as described, you may find that your energy and attention are focused there. Your muscles may start to tighten, energetically "crowding" the client. Now, relax. Let your shoulders sink. Feel your feet on the floor, your contact with the chair. This has the effect of diffusing the intensity of your focus. The most helpful attitude is that of the observer: interested, yet not personally invested. This gives space to the client. The tissue has freedom to move any way that is beneficial.

Your intention is to be helpful: to be aware and present with any change that occurs. Theoretically, the frontal bone should move forward as it releases, directly outward from the face. In actuality, the following may be indications of a good release: a feeling of greater space inside, a rhythm that is fuller and wider, and a feeling of relaxation and ease.

Usually, you will feel a variety of sensations and movements. You may feel pulsation of energy, or a movement forward that is restricted at one point. You may become aware of any of the signs of therapeutic release. Completion is signaled by a return of easy movement, by a sense of space and greater freedom. Gently but clearly, withdraw your contact, lifting your hands away from the forehead.

The Upper Sides of the Skull: The Parietal Bones

The squamous suture between the temporal and parietal bones, forming a partial circle above and behind the ears, is unique. The edges of the bones meet on a diagonal, so the temporal bone overlaps the parietal. In the traditional release procedure, we first hold the parietal bones in as the craniosacral rhythm pushes the temporal bones outward. From about the same finger position, we then lift in a superior direction, that is, toward the top of the head.

At the frontal bone, we assisted in establishing flexibility along all its sutures, including the coronal suture, between the frontal and parietal bones. Our goal here is to assist the body in establishing flexibility along the squamous suture, with the temporal bones, and along the lambdoid suture, with the occiput (the back of the head). As the dura mater relaxes along these sutures, it may influence the falx cerebri. Thus, the inner fold of membrane beneath the sagittal suture can also release constriction.

Resting your forearms on the table, place your hands, palms inward, at the sides of the client's head. Bringing your fingers just behind and above the ears, explore the surface as you slide them upward (toward the top of the head). Find the squamous suture, just above the ears. Exploring further, palpate the slight roughness or ridges on the sides of the skull, above the suture, near the curve of the parietal bone as it forms the top of the skull.

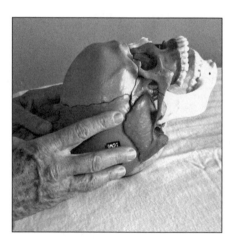

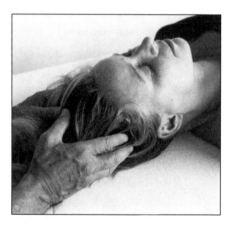

Figure 39a. Finger Positions on the Parietal Bones. The fingers are placed on the parietals, behind the coronal suture with the frontal bone, and above the squamous sutures with the temporal bones. (See also figure 36.)

Figure 39b. Hands in Place for the Parietal Release. The fingers of each hand contact the parietal bones on each side of the head. The touch is high, near the rounded curve at the upper side of the skull. There the therapist may feel small ridges in the bone, caused by muscle attachments from the mandible.

This is the contact area for this release: above the ears and the squamous suture, just below the curve of parietal bone to the top of head. You assure yourself that you are behind the frontal bone by staying just above the ears, on the back portion of the skull.

With your finger pads on the parietal bones, follow the craniosacral rhythm: bones and fingers moving inward, outward, inward. When you are confident of the rhythm, softly hold the parietal bones inward as the rhythm pushes outward. This holding is more by intention and touch than by the use of muscle. Stabilize the parietal bones, holding them inward with your finger pads while the rhythm continues for two cycles, a half minute or less. Then ease your touch, remaining lightly in contact.

Again, palpate the craniosacral rhythm for two or three cycles. The parietal bones are usually free to enter a release process that is similar for many of the bones of the cranium. Continue to touch lightly, but bring your energy from your hands into your body. Let your attention be broad rather than focused narrowly on the parietals.

The important factor is your presence, with respect for the amazing process you are a part of. Follow and work with the indications of release.

You may feel a hesitation on one side or the other. As restrictions ease, greater freedom of movement is restored along the squamous suture with the temporal bones, and along the lambdoid suture with the occiput. As the parietal bones release, the dura mater is affected as it extends around the base of the cranial vault and down the dural tube.

As you continue gently in contact, in tune with the client's body, you may sense restriction or ease in the neck and shoulders. This is more likely in later sessions as you gain experience.

Whether you sense a full release along each suture of the parietal bones, or merely some signs of therapeutic release, disengage after a few minutes. Gently yet clearly lift your hands away from your client's head.

The Floor of the Vault: The Sphenoid

The sphenoid is chiefly an internal bone, connecting the frontal, temporal, and occipital bones to form the floor of the cranial vault. At each side, the greater wings of the sphenoid curve upward to form an outer surface

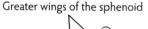
Greater wings of the sphenoid

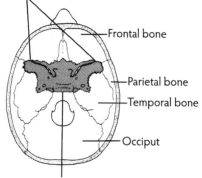

Frontal bone

Parietal bone

Temporal bone

Occiput

Joint of sphenoid with base of occiput

Figure 40. The Floor of the Cranial Vault. A cutaway view, looking down within the cranial vault. The sphenoid forms a unique joint with the base of the occiput. A pad of cartilage at this point allows a rocking motion between these bones at the inner floor of the cranial vault. (See also figure 62 in chapter 8.)

at the temples. We contact the greater wings of the sphenoid beneath the musculature at the temples.

The sphenoid plays a central role in the structure of the head. It articulates with every other bone in the cranial vault, and influences the motion of the facial bones. Major nerves to the eyes, the cheeks, the gums, and the palate pass through openings in the sphenoid. Restrictions in the connective tissue around the sphenoid can impinge on these nerves and affect their functioning.

The sphenoid forms a special joint with the occiput, the sphenobasilar synchondrosis. A pad of cartilage separates the posterior portion of the sphenoid from the base of the occiput. This cushion of absorbent and flexible tissue, deep in the cranium, allows a unique rocking motion at this joint.

In the early days of craniosacral therapy, it was thought that any restriction of the sphenoid could be attributed to an irregularity at this joint. However, this view ignores the special position of the sphenoid. Touching every other bone, it is like a keystone within the cranium. Irregularity of movement in any other cranial bone will be communicated to the sphenoid. Furthermore, the bones of the cranial base respond to constrictions and imbalance within the body. These reach upward from pelvis and torso, shoulders and neck by way of muscle and connective tissue. Thus, the release of constriction and irregular motion of the sphenoid may interact with tissue and joints throughout the body.

The traditional sphenoid release, though designed for the sphenobasilar synchondrosis, works equally well for this broader concept. There are two parts to the procedure, thought of as compression and decompression. In the first, the sphenoid bone moves toward the occiput, compressing the cartilage at its base. This acts as an initial clearing of energy foci or restrictions along its joints with the temporal bones and the occiput. Paradoxically, moving in the direction of compression relieves the soft connective tissue that has been holding the bones in compression.

In the second part of the procedure, the sphenoid moves forward, away from temporal bone and occiput, toward its sutures with the frontal and with the bones of the mouth and face. The effect of these two moves is to "exercise" the connective tissue at all of the sutures of the sphenoid. This movement allows the sphenoid to feel and reassess the condition of its connection to the other bones of the cranial vault.

Resting your forearms on the table, raise your hands to the sides of the client's head. Bring your thumbs to the temples and let your fingers touch where they are comfortable. The little finger will usually be able to reach the occiput.

If the span of your hand is not wide enough to contact both the occiput and the temple, then let the other fingers rest where they are comfortable. Your thumb pads maintain contact with the greater wings of the sphenoid at the temples.

As cerebrospinal fluid is produced, the cranial vault expands, pushing the sphenoid downward, moving the greater wings downward, toward the client's body.

As cerebrospinal fluid is absorbed, the cranial vault contracts, drawing the sphenoid upward. The greater wings move upward, toward the top of the head, toward bregma, the point at the junction of the coronal and sagittal sutures.

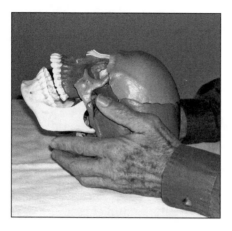

Figure 41a. Finger Positions
on the Sphenoid.

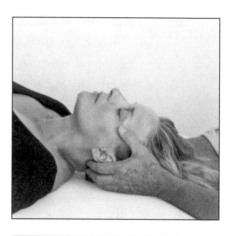

Figure 41b. Hands in Place
for the Sphenoid Release.

The hands lightly contact each side of the head, so that the sides of the thumbs comfortably touch the temples (just behind the corner of each eye). Here, muscle fibers cover the greater wings of the sphenoid on each side of the head. The fingers touch the head while the little fingers curl under to the occiput. The direction of release is initially in the posterior direction, toward the occiput and the back of the head. In the second stage, the sphenoid moves anteriorly, toward the frontal bone. (See also figure 64b in chapter 8.)

Attend to the craniosacral rhythm moving the sphenoid down, toward the body, drawing the sphenoid up, toward bregma. Down and returning, or up and returning: a regular rhythm of the greater wings of the sphenoid.

Follow the rhythm, observing regularity and inconsistencies.

For the first part of the release, use your imagination to suggest a movement back, toward the occiput and the temporal bones. The motion is almost directly downward toward the table.

As your thumb pads meet the sphenoid, using a light touch, bring your awareness to your posture and physical ease. Let your hands, arms, and shoulders be at ease. From your center, as if from a slight distance, observe and follow any motion of the sphenoid back toward the base of the occiput. You may occasionally find it helpful to reposition your thumbs.

The motion of the sphenoid may be uneven and gradual. As it moves back toward its juncture with the base of the occiput, membranes that may have been restricting it are able to ease up, to relax, to release. Tensions along the border with other cranial bones are stirred up; they hold, and let go.

Continue while you have a sense of movement and release. Continue with awareness, respect for this process, and light touch. When the motion is quiet, this part of the release is complete. Now visualize a movement of the sphenoid forward, in the direction of the frontal bone, making space where it joins the base of the occiput.

This movement may also be uneven and gradual. The greater wings of the sphenoid sometimes appear to veer to one side or the other. Maintain awareness, respect for the intention of the body as the release unfolds, and light touch. As the sphenoid moves forward, it activates other areas of restriction in the soft tissue. Rigidified tissue is able to return to a more functional balance between holding and relaxation.

Continue until there is a sense of quiet between thumb pads and sphenoid. Follow the renewed rhythm for a few cycles. Often it will feel fuller and easier. Then lightly and clearly lift your hands away from the client's head.

The Lower Sides of the Skull: The Temporal Bones

The temporal bone houses the ear canal and hearing apparatus and plays host to the external structure of the ear. The sense mechanism for balance is located deep in the temporal bone, within the inner ear. The temporal bone also provides the joint for the lower jaw, just in front of the ear canal. The important functions of hearing, balance, and chewing are performed more effectively when the rhythmic movement of the temporal bones are in phase, or synchronous.

Through muscle attachments and the temporomandibular joint, the lower jaw exerts tremendous leverage on the temporal bone. Habitual clenching or grinding of the teeth may affect the flexibility and alignment of these bones. Clenching of the teeth at a time of powerful, unpleasant emotion may result in the imprinting of emotion and a state of tension on muscle and connective tissue.

Problems of alignment of upper and lower teeth and pain or restriction in using the jaw involve a complex of bones, connective tissue, and joints. Key among them is the temporal bone, its sutures with other bones, and all of its muscle and ligament connections.

The temporal bone joins the parietal, occipital, and sphenoid among the cranial bones. In our work so far we have assisted in the release of restrictions along the squamous suture with the parietal bone and restrictions along the sutures surrounding the sphenoid.

Our goals in working with the temporal bone are to ease restrictions around its sutures and to assist synchronous movement between the bones.

There are three forms of release in this region. The ear pull technique is the most widely used specifically for the temporal bone. It stimulates a general release of restrictions along all the sutures with other bones. Because it helps restore freedom of movement in every dimension, it usually also encourages synchronous movement between the temporal bones.

Both the mastoid release and the three-finger technique address synchronous movement. They are often more effective for fine-tuning than for coping with major restrictions in the sutures and connective tissue.

A finger of the temporal bone (the petrous part) reaches into the cranial base between the occiput and the sphenoid. When we address the temporal bone, we are assisting in the easing of restrictions through this important region of the cranial base. In particular, the hand position for the mastoid release reaches both the occiput and the temporal bones. For a beginning study, the mastoid release is included here. Later, as you repeat full therapy sessions, this position flows well just after the atlanto-occipital release.

The Ear Pull Release

The cartilage of the outer ear is firmly anchored to the temporal bone. Thus, it acts as the handle by which we sense movement and assist release in a lateral (outward) direction. With forearms resting on the table, place the fingers of each hand behind the ears of your client. Place the thumb of each hand in the front of each ear, almost in the ear canal, and grasp the ear between your thumb and fingers. You are making a firm contact with each ear, but not pulling or exerting force.

When you are in position, bring your awareness to your posture and comfort. While making physical contact, always respect the space of your client. You are in your center, observing. Be open to any movement or energetic manifestation. You may sense the craniosacral rhythm. There are two components to its movement. With production and absorption of cerebrospinal fluid, the cranial vault expands and contracts, moving the temporal bones outward and inward.

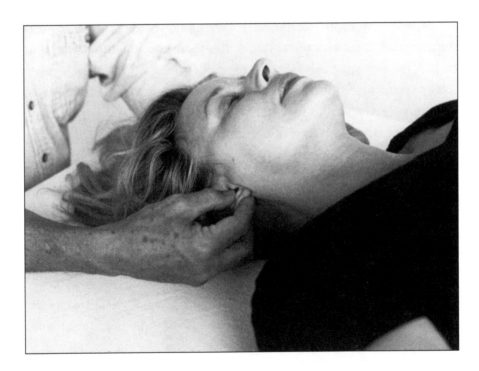

Figure 42. The Ear Pull Release. The fingers of each hand grasp the ear, holding it softly but firmly. Three fingers are behind the ear; the thumb holds inside at the ear canal. The direction of release is on a diagonal, to the side and back.

Holding the ear, you may also sense the second component of the rhythm, a rotation. As the cranial vault expands, the upper part of the temporal bone rotates forward, returning toward the occiput on each contraction.

Initially, attune yourself to the rhythm or other motions that appear. Visualize movement on a diagonal, both outward and back (lateral and posterior). This release follows the direction of the petrous part of the temporal, the finger of bone between sphenoid and occiput. The movement is gradual. Follow it with your intention rather than using force. The lateral motion aids the temporal bone in regaining space along its sutures with the occiput and the parietal bones. The posterior movement helps relieve constriction along the sutures with the sphenoid and the occiput.

The ear pull technique does not stress and stretch the outer ear. With light touch, you signal your intention, then continue to the side and back as the temporal bone responds. You may experience release and hesitation, as with the other cranial bones. Maintain your intention and your patience. Note any signs of therapeutic release. When the release is effective, you will sense a smoothness and synchronization of the movement on both sides.

This is a repetition of attention to some of these sutures, from new directions. Seeking to relieve areas of impacted energy and stress along the suture and in the dura mater, we bring our presence and touch to the cranial vault from one direction, then another.

When you are satisfied that the release is complete, gently disengage. You may then go on to the mastoid and three-finger releases or move directly to the mandible.

The Mastoid Release

Locate the mastoid process, the rounded knob close behind the client's ear. Now place your hands, palms up, on the table on each side of the client's head. Slide them behind the occiput and the neck so that you cradle the head, with each thumb pad on the mastoid process. Your fingers can cross beneath the neck in any way that is mutually comfortable.

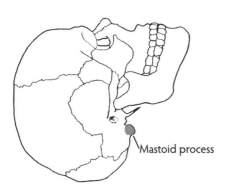

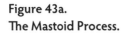

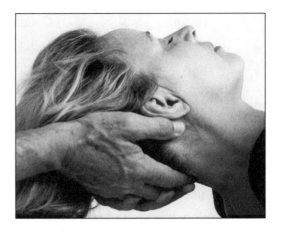

Figure 43a.
The Mastoid Process.

Figure 43b. Hands in Place
for the Mastoid Release.

The hands cradle the head from behind, but do not lift. (The head has been raised
for this illustration.) The thumb of each hand contacts the mastoid process, a
rounded knob on the temporal bone behind each ear. The craniosacral rhythm can
be felt pressing the thumbs outward and returning inward.

As cerebrospinal fluid is produced, your thumb will be pushed outward
by the mastoid process, returning inward as the fluid is absorbed. Sense the
craniosacral rhythm at the mastoid process: pushing outward, returning
inward with each cycle.

Assess the quality of the rhythm. Are the two sides synchronous, moving together? Is the outward motion as strong as the inward motion?

You will often notice variations from a smooth and balanced rhythm.
To employ the traditional release procedure, choose the side that is weaker,
or slower on the inward portion of the cycle. With a light touch, hold
that weaker or slower side stable for two cycles, monitoring the rhythm
with the other hand.

Let the rhythm return on both sides. Then hold in the other side for
two cycles. Let the rhythm return to both sides. Follow it and assess. Is
the rhythm synchronous and even?

Continue with the thumbs lightly monitoring the mastoid processes. This traditional procedure gives a feeling for the movement of the temporal bones. As you gain more experience and sensitivity, you will find that the temporal bones enter a release process without prompting by the therapist. Merely remain present and aware, following with interest the variations of motion and energy. Often toward the end of the process there is a period of quiet. This is followed by a rhythmic return that is synchronous, full, and free.

In the treatment outline in appendix 1, the mastoid release is placed immediately after the atlanto-occipital release. Your hands can move easily to a position cradling the occiput. You can sense along the dural tube. Then, move your thumbs into position on the mastoid processes.

The Three-finger Technique

Locate the mastoid process as described above. You will place your ring finger here.

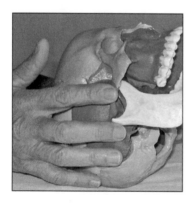

Figure 44a. Three Finger Positions.

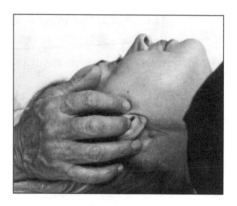

Figure 44b. Hands in Place for the Three-finger Technique.

On each side of the head, the index finger is placed on the zygomatic arch, just in front of ear canal; the middle finger is placed directly in the ear canal; and the fourth finger rests on the mastoid process behind the ear. The craniosacral rhythm can be felt with the second and fourth fingers as the temporal bone rotates in a small arc around the middle finger.

Locate the zygomatic arch. It is a ridge that extends from the ear canal horizontally to the cheek. Place your index finger on the arch, close to the ear canal.

With the index finger on the zygomatic arch near the ear and the fourth finger on the mastoid process, stabilize your hand by placing the middle finger lightly in the opening of the ear canal.

You may sense more than one component of the craniosacral rhythm. Locate the component that seems to rotate the temporal bone, so that your index finger moves toward the chin as your fourth finger moves away. Then both return, rotating back.

Assess the degree to which these rotating movements on each side of the client's head are synchronous. In addition, notice whether the strength of the cycle is as strong in each direction of rotation.

Choose one side and stabilize it by holding the temporal bone in place with your index and fourth finger while monitoring the rhythm with the other hand. Use a light touch. After two cycles ease your touch and monitor both sides.

Then repeat the process on the other side. After two cycles, release.

Let your hands remain in place for awhile, monitoring both sides until they resume a uniform, improved rhythm. Gently release.

The Lower Jaw: The Mandible

With the mouth, and the functioning of the mandible, we obtain nourishment and express ourselves both verbally and physically. If the temporomandibular joint is constricted or painful, then any or all of those natural functions may be impaired. Like the pelvic floor, the mandible is complex in its variety of functions and the emotions associated with each of them.

Muscles and fascia in the shoulders and in the neck reach upward to the occiput and the temporal bones. Any constrictions there may influence the temporomandibular joint. Thus, it is helpful to have addressed these areas as discussed in the previous chapter.

The muscles used in chewing reach upward on each side of the head. Thus, the action of the mandible can exert great pressure on the frontal,

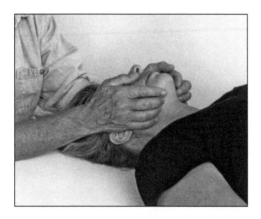

Figure 45. Releasing the Mandible: Compression. The fingers of each hand reach around the mandible to contact it along its lower edge. The ideal direction of movement is superior, as the jaw moves upward on each side, into its joints with the temporal bones.

parietal, and temporal bones. If this pressure is uneven, then these bones are repeatedly pulled asymmetrically. Up to now, we have addressed each of these cranial bones individually.

Rest your forearms or elbows on the table and place your hands along the sides of the client's face. Bring the fingers of each hand to the lower jaw, lightly holding. The fingertips can curl around the lower edge. The aim is to make contact yet maintain a soft touch.

Now bring your awareness inside. Feel the pressure of the chair supporting you; feel your feet resting on the floor. As you maintain presence, giving space to the client, the body tissue often begins to realign itself. Observe and follow. You may notice motion in almost any direction, and any of the signs of release. The client may notice a relaxation in the jaw, the neck, or even the pelvis. During this process, monitor your body, returning to center and ground, returning to a more comfortable posture. Continue in touch for a few minutes, until there is a sense of quiet and completion. Then bring your hands away.

The more traditional approach is to release compression or imbalance at the temporomandibular joint in two stages. In the first, we go in the direction of compression by holding under the body of the mandible and following upward, toward the joint. In the second stage, we hold the body of the mandible at its sides and follow downward, decompressing the joint.

For this two-step procedure, rest your elbows on the table and place your hands along the sides of the client's face as described above. Now, curl your fingers around the lower edge of the mandible. Let your fourth finger find the notch near the posterior angle.

Imagine the mandible moving upward, into its joint with the temporal bone. This is the direction of compression, of muscle contraction and shortening. The goal is to relieve the stress of overworked muscle and connective tissue. Follow with your intention any components of motion in this direction.

After sensations of movement, hesitation, and release, you will sense quietness in the mandible. Release your contact and slide your fingers to the side of the jaw, just above the edge. In particular, make contact with the swelling of muscle at the corner, just above the notch.

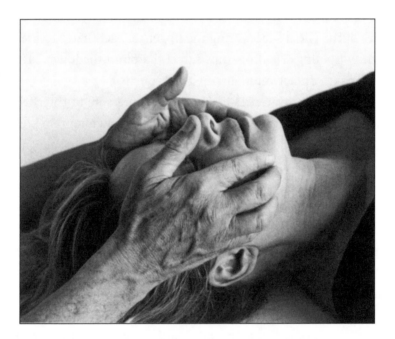

Figure 46. Releasing the Mandible: Decompression. The fingers of each hand touch the body of the mandible along its sides, just above the lower edge. The direction of movement is inferior, following the jaw away from its joint with the temporal bone.

Pressing in slightly to maintain a firm touch, imagine motion downward, away from your position.

Maintain your touch and awareness as you notice hesitation, movement, alternating of energy from side to side, and release. Our goal is to assist a release process that brings a softening of tissue and greater range of motion equally to each side. You can maintain a firmness of intent even as you remain in contact with a light touch.

When the motion has rested and there is a sense of quiet, gently bring your hands away.

You may consider this the completion of the session. However, many therapists enjoy using the following still point procedure at the end of each session.

The Occiput: The CV-4 and the Still Point

Up to this point, we have addressed the occiput in relation to other bones: the atlas, the sphenoid, and the temporal. This procedure works directly with the occiput, though with the intention of reaching beyond it, into the brain's fourth ventricle. (See figure 2 in chapter 1, and figure 52 in chapter 7.)

At times during the process of therapeutic release, the craniosacral rhythm appears to stop. This natural occurrence has come to be called a *still point*. When the rhythm returns, it is usually smoother and stronger.

Because of the apparent beneficial effects of this period of rest, Sutherland and his followers developed methods of inducing a still point by holding a part of the body and dampening the cycle of the craniosacral rhythm. This can be done most readily at the ankles and at the occiput. If the rhythm is temporarily suspended early in a session, some of the minor irregularities may disappear.

The CV-4 technique induces a still point by compressing the occiput behind the fourth ventricle of the brain. In addition to strengthening and smoothing the craniosacral rhythm, this procedure may be helpful in the release of compression around the occipital sutures. Your practice up to this point has prepared you for the delicacy of touch used in the still point.

The hand position involves placing the hands together, palms up, with fingers overlapping. Bring the tips of the thumbs together. This causes the soft pad at the thumb's base to turn upward. Try this with your hands.

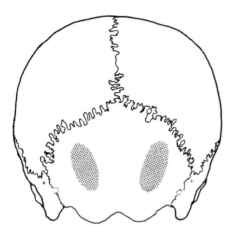

Figure 47. CV-4 Points on the Occiput. Shading at each side illustrates the general area of the occiput that is supported by the soft pads at the base of the thumbs. The area contacted is clear of the sutures and below the external occipital protuberance.

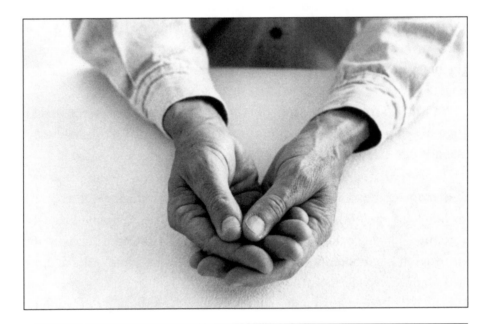

Figure 48. Hand Position for the Still Point. Lay the fingers of one hand across the fingers of the other. Then touch the thumb tips together. This provides a foundation for the client's occiput, which will rest on the fleshy pads covering the first metacarpal at the base of the thumbs.

With this arrangement, the table supports the hands. The fleshy, rounded area at the base of the thumbs is exposed to provide a resting place for the client's occiput.

To discover the target area on yourself, place the fingers of both hands on the back of your head. Find the sensitive point at lambda, the meeting place of the sagittal and lambdoid sutures, just above the occipital prominence. Now follow the lambdoid sutures down and outward on a diagonal. The suture passes through a flattened area between the mastoid process and the muscle attachments at the back of the occiput.

This roughly lambda-shaped, triangular area describes the occiput. The fleshy base of your thumbs will support the client's head at the wide base of the occiput. It is important to be on the occiput, away from the sensitive sutures.

The most straightforward way to place your hands is to form the proper position, then slip them into place when the client raises his or her head. When you place your hands, feel free to ask your client to raise his or her head until you are confident that you are supporting the occiput only. Modify your hand position for relative comfort.

In carefully placing the hands, the shoulders and arms may tighten. Take time to let the shoulders drop, the muscles ease. Maintain your center. You will sense the occiput swelling outward against your support, then returning, with each cycle of the craniosacral rhythm. Follow the rhythm for several cycles, noticing variations between the sides and in the cycle itself.

The traditional approach is to follow the cycle inward and hold. This holding is as much with intention and presence as it is through any pressure of the hands. In fact, presence and respect for the inner process is far more powerful than any level of manipulative pressure.

When you feel ready, move in with the inward cycle of the rhythm and lightly hold. Be aware and respectful of the rhythm, yet persist in your intention to stabilize the occiput inward.

As with other procedures, you may experience a release of energy: heat, electricity, pain. Practitioners often sense energy moving in a "ping-pong" effect from side to side.

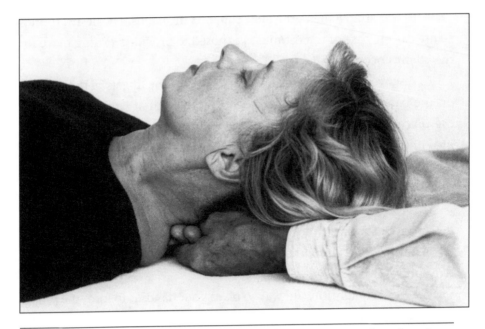

Figure 49. Hands in Place for the Still Point. The occiput rests on the soft pads at the base of thumbs. Take care to support the occiput and not put pressure on the lambdoid suture to each side. The craniosacral rhythm can be felt pressing the occiput outward against the hands, and returning inward.

The rhythm may stop briefly, then return. Merely stay with it, observing, present and respectful.

When all motion and indications of therapeutic release have become still, continue holding for a few seconds. Then relax your touch and intent while keeping your hands in almost the same position. Experience the quality of the motion as the rhythm returns. It may be tentative at first and then gain momentum. Continue with your hand position until the cycle has stabilized. How does the rhythm compare to what you observed before the still point? What has been your client's experience?

Completion

A full craniosacral session includes the listening stations, the releases of the body, and the cranial releases. The completion phase that follows is as important as the release procedures. Completion provides for a return to ordinary conscious awareness and integration of physiological shifts. The role of the practitioner includes signaling to your client that it is time to return, remaining present, and giving space.

The client is often in a very deep state of relaxation at the end of the session. The energetic and physical adjustments that have intensified during the session may continue for hours or days. Yet it is now time for the client to return to an ordinary state of consciousness. You may signal this by touch and with words. I find it helpful to move from the head to the body, briefly touching as in the listening stations. I gently rock the legs and squeeze the feet with a little massage. This signals a change in tempo and helps bring awareness to the body and the ground after so much focus on the upper body and head.

I make this contact clear and precise, then let go. It is important to give space, allowing the client to feel whatever is occurring inside. This is not a time to prolong contact, embrace, or begin a long conversation. Part of the transition and integration for the client involves getting up from the massage table and taking a few steps. As therapist, I remain present but stand apart as the client reconnects with the ground and experiences the body anew.

During this transition, the therapist's physical presence is reassuring and supportive. So remain in the room until the client is clearly back to an ordinary state of consciousness. Then is the time for final words and a touch or embrace.

Chapter 4

Beyond the Technique: Integration, Assessment

The listening stations, the releases of the body, and the cranial releases constitute a full session of craniosacral therapy. This step-by-step procedure forms a standard protocol that touches many crucial points of the body, places that may manifest learned responses such as pain, limited range of motion, or restriction of function. Even the beginning practitioner can help people suffering from these symptoms through a careful and sensitive application of the craniosacral protocol.

Through repetition of this protocol, through giving and receiving sessions, the therapist's inner awareness grows. He or she learns in the mind and in the body how this work helps, how these procedures operate between client and therapist. The client also learns, with mind and body, what to expect and how to benefit from craniosacral sessions.

Therefore, my recommendation to new practitioners is to do as many complete sessions as possible, to learn through doing. Watch and nourish the development of these skills and attitudes: the ability to touch clearly yet softly; the awareness of self as well as client; the capability to listen to the direction of the body itself; the attitude of respect and awe toward the process in which we are involved; the ability to remain grounded and centered while giving space to the client. Experience the pleasure of being a part of these wonderfully effective processes.

Integration

After discovering craniosacral work, many body therapists ask: "How do I integrate it into my present work?" Many bodyworkers who offer massage, Shiatsu, or reflexology would like to know how to blend craniosacral into one of these sessions.

Many therapists begin to add a part of what they have learned into their usual session. However, I believe this is a mistake. To truly learn craniosacral therapy, to realize fully its potential, it is important to offer full sessions. Offering full sessions, separate from any other familiar modality, the therapist learns from within. He or she learns more and more about the quality of touch, about the release process, about connections and patterns in the body.

Thus, this work is first integrated into the inner knowing of the therapist. This is important because craniosacral is much more than a set of procedures. Craniosacral therapy combines a philosophy of healing with the unfolding of personal qualities and skills.

It is the repeated practice of these skills, qualities, and practical philosophy that leads to an inner integration, an inner sense of what this is about.

As that happens, the integration of modalities will begin to occur naturally and spontaneously. The therapist will find herself or himself blending touch and procedures from many sources, without effort or conscious planning. This produces the most effective integration of therapy modalities.

Assessment

Assessment is the process of becoming aware of the patterns of flow and constriction manifested by the client. The attitude of assessment leads the practitioner to look over the whole before beginning at a part and to keep the view broad rather than narrowly focused.

In the first chapter of this book, the listening stations were presented as a useful beginning to the session and to the assessment process. Through touching, "watching," and "listening" at these points from ankles to head, we are able to observe indications of flow or concentration, as well as the changing quality of the craniosacral rhythm.

When we palpate the two sides of the body, a lack of symmetry in the craniosacral rhythm indicates an asymmetrical constriction in muscles or connective tissue. A symmetrical but generally constricted rhythm indicates to us a more general constriction of tissue. Such generalized constriction usually fragments the transmission of both fluid and energy in the body. It interferes with cohesive movement among body parts.

The quality of body energy is another useful sign of freedom or restriction in body function. However, it is not as easily defined or described as the craniosacral rhythm. Various healing practitioners have developed their own vocabularies to talk about body energy. Often they perceive and describe it differently, and release or treat it in a wide assortment of styles. The common theme is that experienced bodyworkers or therapists often begin to "see" more than meets the unpracticed eye. They may see colors, receive physical sensations, have images of inner organs appear in the mind's eye, or simply move the hands to a place that seems to beckon. These are natural capabilities. However, we often ignore them in modern society. As you practice craniosacral therapy, you will begin to notice the reawakening of a broader awareness. That may be soon, it may be later. It will probably change form as you gain more experience.

There is no special vocabulary to use, no proper set of signals to notice. The secret of awakening your awareness is to become increasingly conscious of your own subtle perceptions and intuitions. Anything you notice is the "right" thing at this moment. Often, the craniosacral rhythm will not be the major focus. What is important is to attend to whatever the body is manifesting, and to let go of concepts or learning that restrict how or what you perceive. In this way, you are opening yourself to continuous development of insight and skill.

The growing awareness and sensitivity within you springs from an inner dialog between client and therapist. This dialog, below the level of consciousness, can find many forms of verbal expression. Each of us perceives the other from within the context of our personal life and experience. Your experience may be different from the client's, and it may be different from some deeper "reality." Its function is to alert you, beckon you. The images and sensations each of us finds most meaningful are not accurate in a scientific sense, but appropriate and useful personally. Therefore, be open to differing viewpoints, differing modes of experience and expression.

Assessment may also involve putting into words those impressions and assumptions that have risen from below conscious awareness. Finding words helps communication and learning for the practitioner, between practitioner and client, and among practitioners. If I formulate an impression of what I perceive before the session, then I learn of the reality and meaning of my observations as I proceed. I learn to correct my impressions and assumptions, and to apply that to future sessions.

In describing my experience, I use ordinary language. I attempt to describe without interpretation or judgment. This leaves me open to new information and to new possibilities. See appendix 2 for some further thoughts on the use of words in our work.

In part 2, presumably after some months experience, we will again discuss touch and assessment. At this time, we will go into more detail, based on your greater experience in this work.

Combining Assessment and Treatment

Though we often think of the listening stations as assessment and the releases as treatment, there is no clear dividing line. From the first moments of contact, both are occurring. Client and therapist are getting to know one another (assessing) from the first words, the first glance, the first touch. Likewise, the body begins responding. With only a light touch to the ankles, for example, the craniosacral rhythm may pause, the breathing may change, the client may visibly relax as muscle tone changes throughout the body. Throughout the listening stations, changes take place in the flow or concentration of body energy. The signs of therapeutic release accompany the therapist as she or he moves up the body. Thus, the listening stations clearly form a part of the treatment phase of the session.

Likewise, as the therapist proceeds into the releases, he or she will work most effectively through keeping open the attitude of assessment. The attitude of assessment reminds us to keep a broad view and an open mind, receptive to changing patterns and possibilities as the session progresses. Furthermore, it reminds us to give space to the client, as we, the therapists, retain our own space.

I keep a broad view. As I touch any specific place, I attempt to remain aware of the whole body, to remain open to any indications that I may notice near to where I touch, or at a distance. I do not move to every place that catches my attention. Rather, I recognize that each person's body has its own set of connections, and I observe these unique connections as they manifest themselves. I stand in awe of the manner in which the body can take advantage of the slightest touch or energy to heal itself when given the space and support.

I keep my mind open to the unexpected. I recognize that with each client, I touch a unique individual with a unique pattern of constrictions, and a unique path of unfolding and release. Firm notions of what will help or what this person needs interfere. They crowd the space, limit possibilities. Keeping an open mind communicates a sense of space. The body/being on the table senses that it is truly free to move in any direction that is helpful. Because I am continually surprised and delighted by what happens, the sessions remain alive and interesting to me.

I give space, physical and mental, to the client. Often the intensity and subtlety of the session entices the therapist. I may find myself closing my eyes, focusing very narrowly, and leaning toward the client. The client can feel pressured, crowded, although my touch remains light. Therefore, I repeatedly return my attention to my own body, to my energy. I stand or sit comfortably, body erect and balanced within itself, energy free and flowing. If the work is becoming intense, I again center myself, regain contact with the ground, and regain my personal space even as I touch. This results in a greater sense of freedom for the client and comfort for me as the therapist, even as I maintain close contact.

Keeping a broad view includes remaining aware of myself. I am aware of my energy and my posture. In addition, I attempt to develop an awareness of my personal pains and constrictions, physical and emotional. This subtle work has the power to uncover layers of hurt and loss in both the therapist and the client. If I am aware of what is mine, if I have acknowledged and accepted it, then I am able to be calm and confident as the client's pain comes to the surface. Because of my personal experience, I can support the client on his or her journey without the need to interfere or control. I can allow the client to experience his or her pain, and respect the client's personal path toward release.

Responding to Symptoms

Many sessions begin with the client's report of pain or restriction. Usually these symptoms are localized in a few places in the client's body. The listening stations and the session itself broaden the picture, revealing a larger assortment of restrictions than reported by the client. The reason for this is that most of us have the ability to suppress our awareness of pain or dysfunction. Despite injury or trauma, we have the urge to get on with day-to-day life, to look beyond our hurts and limitations. We tend to suppress body awareness until, with continued stress or repeated injury, the body sends very strong signals. These strong signals become symptoms that urge us to pay attention to the body, ultimately bringing us to therapy.

However, as therapists, we want to pay attention to the whole body, to address the broader pattern, rather than merely the strongest symptom. The listening stations and the releases provide a treatment protocol that encourages us to do that: to balance our time and energy, observation and response over many areas of the body. The sensitivity that we develop through repeated practice guides us in our timing and emphasis.

Placing the hands at the points of greatest pain may help the therapist to sense this pain more immediately, and to sense some of its connections with other parts of the body. However, often it is not helpful to remain at a very painful place waiting for releases. Such prolonged direct contact may only intensify the symptom. Generally, we encourage the release of severe pain by placing the hands near the painful place or on places that appear connected. This helps the surrounding tissue and organs to reestablish flow and communication through the constricted point.

It is always helpful to work with the whole body, no matter what the symptom or complaint. When we touch other points, points that seem less important, we often discover that release there contributes greatly to the relief of the symptom. Sometimes these connections appear during the listening stations; sometimes we discover them later. At other times, a distant release may be a total surprise to both therapist and client.

The Context of Healing

The healing process begins long before the session and continues after it. It is a process of adjustment through the whole body and person. We touch only for a brief moment in the lifetime of the client. If we respect that process, we work with it, rather than try to overcome or divert it. We recognize that there is wisdom in the body even when that wisdom is not clear to the mind or to our intuitive sensitivity. It is usually more effective to follow the changing pattern throughout the body than to focus on only a few places. The body can more effectively integrate and use a number of small releases rather than one big one. The integration and stabilization of a freer pattern of flow and movement continues for hours or days after the session.

Flexibility

Traditionally, therapists have described very specific directions along which release occurs. These directions spring from an idealized concept of cranial anatomy and the craniosacral rhythm. For simplicity, they tend to view each bone and its sutures independently of the entire matrix of connective tissue.

In reality, we are always dealing with a complex network of freedom and restriction. The pathway to greater ease of function and freedom of movement is unique to each individual. Therefore, it is always important to be sensitive and aware of the signals you are receiving from the client's body. If a release is not working in the direction described, relax, maintain contact, follow what the tissue is trying to do. I have always experienced success when I have stayed with the tissue through all of its movements, even when it does not seem to be moving in the "proper" direction.

Taking Care of the Therapist

Whether you are exploring the craniosacral rhythm through the self-palpation exercises or practicing the listening stations and the releases on a client, I would encourage you to be aware of your own breath, state of relaxation or tension, and physical comfort. This attitude of awareness and care of the self is important for the long-term development of your healing capacity.

The self is a part of the total healing environment around the client. The healthier you are, the more beneficial the total environment.

Care of the self is part of the objectivity that is necessary to develop a comprehensive perception of the situation that involves your client and yourself. Narrowing of focus may initially seem to result in a breakthrough for the client. However, such an apparent improvement may not endure if it does not fit into the wider picture of the client's healing process. Giving space is a far more powerful healing instrument than attempting to force or direct the healing process. Here patience and trust in the whole process are often more beneficial than pushing, or sacrificing self for an immediate, gratifying result.

Caring for the self may mean allowing yourself to get more distance within the treatment, to move your body, or just get a different view of the process. Breathing freely and remaining clear in your own body means that you are continuing to bring to the client and the situation a fresh, resourceful instrument: yourself.

Receiving regular sessions of craniosacral therapy and other forms of bodywork also helps keep you renewed and present in the healing process. The therapist who is present with his or her life energy is the therapist who is involved in his or her own personal process of growth and transformation. Trust in the healing process is affirmed as you experience that process in yourself.

In summary, take care of yourself, both during and outside of sessions.

Aftercare

In releasing long-term restrictions, craniosacral therapy demonstrates to the body's tissue that it can again safely move through a fuller range. Processes of release begin during a session, but these are processes that continue after the session. Often, the tissue will continue to experiment with possibilities of movement, release, and integration for hours or days afterward.

After a full session, the body is more open and vulnerable than before. In responding to the hands of the therapist, the body has let go of natural defenses, defenses that have served it well. After the session, the client is returning to an ordinary state of consciousness, reestablishing groundedness and presence in the here and now.

It is best to avoid stressful situations soon after a session, such as driving in traffic, shopping, and dealing with the demands of other people. After one particularly pleasant session, I got in my car and spent over an hour in heavy rush hour traffic on the way home. I could feel the benefits of the session drain away as tension reestablished itself in my body. When tissue has learned to be ready for trouble, it takes little to trigger the defensive response of tightening, swelling, and pain.

Some rest and retreat are recommended after a session, in proportion to the degree of unwinding that has occurred. Suggest that your client lie on the table for a while or take a gentle walk outdoors before getting in the car or on public transportation. The natural movement of gentle walking out of doors or even sitting quietly in nature can be very beneficial in continuing the reintegration process at every level of consciousness.

On the other hand, natural alertness and simple activity are healthy. As the body moves in walking, it integrates changes that took place in the session. Craniosacral practice induces a very relaxed state, an altered state of consciousness that can be very alluring. If healing implies expanded capacity to function in the actual environment, the here and now, then awakening to ordinary consciousness and activity are part of the process. Again, the goal is to expand consciousness and capability rather than suppress pain and problem areas. With recuperation comes gradual renewed involvement in a full life.

Emotional Release

When deep into release and healing, the client often experiences images, memories, and unusual sensations and emotion. Sometimes these are very powerful. When you are sharing such an intense situation with a client, it is especially important to be aware of your own emotional, mental, and physical responses that may be triggered.

If the client is entering an emotionally laden release, then it is usually safe to assume that this is the appropriate time and place for that to happen. It is safe to assume that the client also has the inner resources to navigate through and benefit from the experience and the release.

My response as practitioner is to remain calmly present and supportive. Often it is sufficient to be there without saying anything. It is wonderful, as a client, to feel supported and to be able to express and experience deep emotion. It is not helpful for the therapist to get involved in this part of the client's experience.

If you wish to use words, then use as light a touch with words as you have learned to use with your hands. A very helpful word is a simple yes, affirming the client's experience. You may simply ask, "Can you tell me something about what you are experiencing?" In addition, you might ask the client to describe an experience or image more fully. Repeat parts of the description to reinforce your presence and attention. Ask for associated colors, feelings, smells, or shapes if the description seems very intellectual. Follow your intuition in this. But keep the intervention minimal.

It is very important to let the client have the experience that he or she is ready for. A light touch, verbally and personally, is as important here as in the cranial releases. There is no need to get all the details or have a logically cohesive story. Seeking more details may stimulate pain rather than healing. When the body itself is at rest, peaceful, and expansive, then the release process is complete. Let go of it and transition with the client to whatever is next.

After an emotional release, how do you assess the experience? Verbalization and emotional expression are usually more intriguing and gratifying to both the therapist and the client. They give the mind more to hold on to and mull over. At times, we tend to judge a session by the excitement expressed.

Yet, physical and biological change is gradual. We are dealing with an entire interconnected being. There is no evidence to indicate that strong emotional releases or gripping stories are more profoundly releasing and renewing than quieter sessions accompanied by clear evidence of therapeutic release.

Memories

At times, there is a coherent and compelling memory or story associated with an emotional release. How true is the story?

My experience suggests that we do not know how to evaluate the validity of the story, no matter how coherent and compelling it is. To get caught up in questioning whether the story or memory really happened is to miss the therapeutic point of the image and experience.

The stories, images, and emotions associated with therapeutic release appear to be part of the individual person's means of coping with a limitation: a limitation that may involve past tissue injury, painful memory, fear, or anxiety.

The "story line" laden with emotion and apparent memory during a release may be a metaphor constructed by the nonconscious self to dramatize and bring to conscious awareness certain crucial issues. To believe or not to believe in the story seems less important than to bring to conscious awareness the issues the story represents. Time and involvement in the life process bring integration and healing.

Physical, Mental, Emotional, or Spiritual?

The inquiring mind creates polarities: conscious and unconscious, matter and spirit, matter and energy, physical and emotional, mental and emotional, religion and science. We have learned to define concepts so that they are exclusive of one another rather than inclusive.

Craniosacral practice explicitly joins physical science and consciousness in its inquiry, method, and explanatory discourse. It treats these as a unity rather than as competing realms. For instance, it views any physiological phenomenon as the manifestation of the physical, the nonconscious, and the conscious acting as a unity.

When we talk of emotional release, it is because the emotion is so apparent. But the emotional release has always occurred in the context of a physical tissue release. Longtime practitioners of craniosacral therapy find themselves also dealing with the spiritual dimension—their own as well as the client's. It seems that although we define these realms distinctly, they exist as a unity within each person. The presence of one dimension is a signal that all are involved.

We solve the problems of the polarities set up by our minds not by further analysis but by deeper awareness and openness to experience.

Healing Energy and Sexual Energy

At times therapist and client find themselves attracted to one another, romantically or sexually. How do these feelings and impulses fit into the context of a healing relationship?

Perhaps it is because of our societal conditioning and our learned way of thinking that we are surprised when this happens. At some place deep within, human energies are not separate, but one. When we are closely involved with another person, it is natural to have feelings of tenderness, affection, or sexual attraction.

It is essential within the therapeutic relationship that the client is free to explore and express what comes up physically and emotionally. The touch and support of the therapist encourage this exploration. At the same time, the therapist needs to be grounded, calm, and respecting of boundaries in order to provide a safe environment for the client to explore.

The therapist's issues of pain and need are often touched within a session. That is why it is so important that she is aware, accepting, and dealing with these issues in herself. When the therapist uses the session to dwell on and express these needs, the environment is no longer safe for the client.

The energy of healing transformation and the energy of sexual expression are both intense manifestations of human energy. Each can be consuming, life changing, exciting, as well as confusing.

Therapy and friendship are different relationships. When two people become intimately involved as friends, then the therapeutic relationship is over. It is extremely difficult for the therapist to remain calm, supportive, objective, and consciously aware of the total situation and also be romantically involved. Love or sex stirs up our deep-rooted expectations, fears, hopes, and demands. In the long term, we work these out with our partner. It is a process of discovery and emergence to new ways of living, loving. Partners are equal, equally discovering, exploring, and sharing.

The therapeutic relationship has allure. The client experiences the therapist at his or her most nurturing, caring, supportive, and effective. It is the nature of the work to be able to be that way for hours at a time. Yet, that is not a fully accurate picture of the therapist. No one is that way all the time.

The therapist experiences the client at his or her most open, vulnerable, brave, eager to get on with life, and willing to share the most personal of intimacies. Again, it is the nature of the process that the client can be that way for an hour with one person. That is not the whole of the client.

The therapeutic process brings these capabilities together for healing, for opening to new life. It is difficult really to know the other person from a therapeutic relationship. Moreover, when we follow the energy or desire to a different expression, then we are making the choice to let go of the therapeutic relationship.

Perhaps other opportunities will open. Perhaps the romantic attraction can grow into a long-term partnership. It is important for both therapist and client to realize the choice they are making if they go in this direction. Neither is a wrong choice. Nevertheless, both parties need to be clear about the implications of such a choice.

Case Examples

Following are examples of work with clients who suffered from a variety of problems.

1. A man in his twenties requested sessions because he was suffering from severe headaches at work and experiencing pain in his lower back. At the beginning of the first session, he described a challenging and rewarding job that required managerial, teaching, and creative skills. He also mentioned that he would be leaving that behind to join his fiancée in another city. Despite his personal qualities and job skills, the relationship sounded somewhat dependent, with him accommodating to her detailed plans for their life together. However, we did not discuss that aspect.

By the second session, the frequency of his headaches had diminished. At the third session, he announced that he had moved out of his fiancée's home and broken off the engagement.

He continued to receive craniosacral sessions periodically for two or three months. His headaches disappeared, and the pain in his lower back was gradually relieved. During that time he found a place to live on his own and became involved in his personal and work life with a new sense of freedom and personal capability.

2. A woman in her thirties sought sessions because of intense pain in her upper back, between the shoulder blades. She operated a small business offering personal care and grooming. During the workday she was either managing the business or bending over her clients.

After two sessions, she reported that the pain had left her upper back and was now in the lower back. "But that's okay, because that's where it started," she said. Within two or three more sessions, the pain had completely left her back. She felt physically more balanced and energetic.

She continued to work as she had before, facing business and personal challenges, perhaps with more confidence, and with no return of physical pain.

3. A woman in her late thirties sought craniosacral therapy to discover its potential. She considered it an aid in exploring her own body, mind, and spirit. Professionally she was a competent organizer, teacher, and body therapist.

She received two full sessions, very much as described in this text. There was almost no discussion during the sessions. For several days after the second session, she felt very sad and kept to herself. During this time, she realized she had been sexually abused as a child. She then took this into therapy with a female therapist and began to reorganize her thinking about her life.

4. A woman in her forties sought help for lower back pain that was almost incapacitating. She had experienced severe back pain before and this reoccurrence scared her.

Her work was very challenging and physically draining. It combined individual counseling, managerial responsibilities, and long hours. It paid well but was not her dream for herself. She was also involved in a rewarding relationship and hoped to be married.

Her body responded well to the first session. Nevertheless, as she moved in preparing to get up from the treatment table, the pain returned and she burst into tears. I urged her to carefully get up, stand, and then move around the room. As she did, the pain subsided.

She returned for several weekly sessions. During the first few weeks, she experienced a reduced level of pain. Over a period of six sessions the chronic pain diminished until she was free of back pain. She continued her work and personal life with greater comfort.

5. A retired man in his late sixties came for craniosacral therapy because of chronic pain in his lower back and right hip. Besides the back pain, he experienced recurrent anxiety that exacerbated the back pain. He also

suffered from polyps in his nasal passages and was considering having them removed surgically.

Over the course of five or six sessions, the back pain was relieved. As he continued receiving sessions he reported that he was becoming aware of the sources of stress in his life, finding ways to cope with anxiety before it took hold of him. He was interested and excited about these developments in his life. During this period, the polyps shrank so much that surgery was no longer recommended.

He continued to do well, and no longer felt the need for sessions. After many months, he again experienced some back pain. He called for an appointment, but was unable to fit it into a busy social and recreational life. Around the same time, his nasal polyps began to be a problem. Later I learned that he obtained medication for the back pain and had the polyps surgically removed.

6. A woman in her seventies experienced pain in her right shoulder. Medical treatments, including cortisone injections, had been ineffective. Craniosacral releases in the shoulder area provided relief after three sessions.

These examples demonstrate that often physical pain is associated with periods of stress or transition in life. A polarizing view might immediately ask, "Is it really physical, or just psychological?" My sense is that the two travel hand in hand, and that no symptom can be reduced to one or the other.

Through this gentle therapy, a person can become quiet and centered and experience new freedom in the body. At the same time, this sense of greater comfort and ease does not just occur in the body tissue, but permeates the whole being as the person begins to make decisions that are more constructive for self.

The second example shows pain and dysfunction retreating to an earlier stage before finally disappearing. At times, we have the capacity not only to ignore the body's message but also to displace it to a more acceptable location. Sometimes we merely deaden our sensitivity to the body. In such instances, healing work will often result in a temporary resurgence of old pain patterns as we listen to the body, give it permission to heal, and then witness the process of release.

Such patterns of pain may show up a day or two after a craniosacral session. They usually build up, peak, and diminish within a few days. At times they occur during the session and last only minutes.

In the third example, the client is pursuing change and renewal in her life. To truly open the self to change is always dangerous to the status quo. When a person is open, there is no guarantee what course will be taken by life events. Yet, I believe such receptiveness is a condition for lasting healing, both for the client and for the therapist.

When a therapist meets such a person, I believe that it is important to be respectful of the client's choices. That client did not return, but sought the support of another therapist. She also decided to process many of her feelings by herself. As far as I have discovered, this has been productive for her.

In the fourth, fifth, and sixth examples, the clients sought help primarily for physical symptoms. In the fourth, preoccupation and a sense of frustration over the back pain had become almost as intense as the pain itself. Centering herself and experiencing pain relief and peace of mind gave the client renewed capacity to cope with the unpleasant aspects of her life.

The man in the fifth example also experienced relief and a new view of his life space and his personal capacities. However, his main goal appeared to have been to get on with life as he had always known it. When symptoms returned he chose medical remedies that offered an immediate reduction of symptoms.

This is an important example. There are always individuals who seem to benefit from craniosacral or some other alternative therapy. Yet, after experiencing improvement, a small setback sends them to a more traditional or a more dramatic form of therapy. This, too, is part of the life experience of the therapist or practitioner.

Part II

·ﾞ¦ﾞ·

Specialized Assessment in Craniosacral Therapy

The basic course presented in the first part of this book provides the therapist with an extremely valuable protocol for a full craniosacral session. This work alone has proven to be immensely helpful to people suffering from chronic pain and restricted movement. Furthermore, the full treatment protocol provides a structure within which the therapist can develop deeper sensitivity and greater skill in the use of these gentle techniques.

Part 2 takes a closer look at many of the skills and attitudes of craniosacral therapy. While many specific procedures are introduced, the main theme is the expansion of your own sensitivity, effectiveness, and joy as a therapist.

We begin with touch. Touch is the key element in all hands-on therapies, and the fundamental means of contact between therapist and client. The quality of a person's touch is an expression of her or his experience and reflects inner qualities.

Touch stimulates a healing process, which we witness in the form of therapeutic release, introduced in chapter 2. Chapter 5 returns to the notion of therapeutic release and considers the process called *unwinding*. Touch and sensitivity to the process of release within the body together constitute the foremost teachers and guides in our work.

The experienced therapist often moves intuitively toward the place of pain or constriction. Chapter 6 explores this process of noticing and responding, which can serve as a guide during the session. This natural capability is enhanced through understanding and practice. Taken alone, this capability may form part of the process of assessment. However, it goes beyond our usual notion of assessment, because it is most useful when it is active and alive throughout the session.

Chapter 7 offers a detailed review of the brain's protective and nourishing environment, the cranial vault.

In chapter 8, we move to specific therapeutic procedures. We will look in greater depth at the cranial base, gaining an enhanced appreciation of its complexity and functioning, and develop broader skills to aid in assisting the return of full functioning.

Moving outward from the cranial vault, chapter 9 presents the bones of the mouth and face, their interrelationship and motions, and the means to assess and release the results of injury.

In the last chapter are some reflections and recommendations to the therapist for using this vast array of knowledge effectively.

Chapter 5

The Art of Touch

Touch is more than the contact of hand to skin. In therapy, touch represents a meeting and interchange between two total individuals. As I reach out to make contact with the client, I am reaching out to discover who and what this is. I feel beyond cloth or skin, to inner body tissue, to muscle and organ, flow and stagnation. I sense freedom and restriction, harmony and pain.

The client attempts through words to describe the pain or restriction, and its origin. The body speaks, too, presenting a broader picture. To the sensitive touch, it reveals a pattern of connections buried below the awareness of the ordinary conscious mind. Muscle and connective tissue, nerves and joints team up to support, protect, and compensate for an injury that has not fully healed. The most obvious symptom may not be the origin of the pain or the key to recovery. Rather, it is often the one place that the body has found a voice to express itself, to call attention to pain that has been suppressed by the determination to get on with a normal life.

Touch is felt by both therapist and client. In reaching out to a client, I also convey qualities of my body, of my inner flow and stagnation, freedom and restriction, harmony and pain.

Touch and Awareness

How do I prepare myself as therapist to sense most effectively what the client is presenting to me, consciously and nonconsciously? How do I maintain clarity so that I know what is coming from the client and what is coming from me? How do I support my body so that I am able to move freely and with fluidity? How do I bring a healing and sacred energy to the session so that each of us may feel lighter and freer after the session?

To begin with my body: I attempt to make clear, definite contact with my hand. I let my arm rest lightly on the client, enhancing contact and easing my muscles. I maintain awareness of each part of my body that is contacting the client.

When I hold my arm upward, off the client, the muscles tighten, the shoulder lifts. That tightness is conveyed to the client. A tension comes between us.

When I focus narrowly on my hand and a small segment of the client's body, I may become so preoccupied that I move unknowingly into an uncomfortable position. Or, I may become so excited by what seems to be happening that I ignore my body comfort. Again, this is communicated to the client's body, as surely as any other aspect of the session. In this work, we communicate by many other channels in addition to ordinary conscious perception. Furthermore, the discomfort I wish to ignore takes a portion of my inner attention. I am not as free, present, or aware as I would be if my body were relaxed. My perceptions are clouded.

My suppression of my pain, my ignoring of my discomfort, are messages that I am sending out even as I am attempting to alleviate the client's pain. It is a confusing message to pass on at this time.

Thus, a fundamental aspect of clear, effective touch is the physical comfort and the continued self-awareness of the therapist.

Study and practice are important aspects of a therapist's preparation and growth. Nevertheless, fundamental to all application of learning and technique is the personal development of the therapist. Inner balance is fundamental to outer balance; inner clarity, to clarity of vision. Sensitivity to the self is a basis for sensitive awareness of what the client is present-ing. Calm, compassionate acceptance of the self is fundamental to calm acceptance of the client's experience.

These personal qualities are always in process; they are a lifetime in development. Yet, they are natural qualities that we all possess to some degree. The therapy session is a forum that draws on and challenges all of my personal qualities. Outside the session, in the quiet spaces of my personal life I am able to reflect on the inner capacities that my interac-tion with the client seems to demand of me. Here is an attempt to express some of these in words.

I Am Present

I bring my attention to this experience, to the here and now. That includes what I perceive of the client's physical and emotional energy, as well as all the thoughts and feelings this situation stimulates in my own conscious-ness. I attempt to balance this presence, so that I am constantly with the client and with myself.

If my mind is repeatedly wandering to other thoughts and ideas, then I am not in the present, and there must be some difficulty remaining in contact with this client. Is it because I am tired, lacking the energy? Or, may it be that some issues stirred up by this situation are difficult for me to acknowledge? On the other hand, am I trying to achieve something in the session that is my goal, my personal issue? It may be triggered by the client's process, but not truly representing the client.

At times, my mind is full of questions, and I'd like to squeeze an answer out of Existence. I may feel inadequate and uncertain about what I am doing. Yet if I am able to be fully present in this experience, I will sense what to do next. I may not know why, I may not have the rational expla-nation I desire, but I will have the direction that I need in this moment.

I Am Centered

I recall my attention and my energy inward. Can I find and feel a center? This helps to reduce the unspoken pressure on the client to perform for the therapist. It gives space. A practical way to recall my center is merely to slightly move my body, to squirm a little or shuffle my feet on the floor. Rather than force my awareness, this draws my awareness inside.

In this context, *center* is not a specific point in my body. Rather, it is a general awareness of the inner self, the inner body.

Often in my life or in a session my thoughts and feelings seem to be pulled outward in many directions. I am wondering if I will succeed; I am thinking of the expectations of my client or someone close to me. If something intense is happening, if the client is crying, in pain, or even full of complimentary comments, I may become preoccupied with that.

All these speculations and preoccupations are a part of my experience, of the here and now. However, they may obscure my perception of the broader context. Quiet, centered energy is the ideal platform for observing all that is going on in a situation. So I attempt to acknowledge what I think, feel, or fear, and to let it be, to return my inner awareness to a place of quiet. I observe and I move from this center.

Anytime I am uncertain, or have been unusually active, I return to this center. I make my next move not from what I have been thinking, or from what the client has been saying, but from this silent inwardness. It may seem consistent with what has preceded. Or it may seem inconsistent. I have grown to have confidence in this movement from an inner sense rather than a movement based on logic and consistency.

At My Center, I Am at Peace

It is a quiet center. It is open and receptive to the total context. This quiet center can perceive subtle nuances. It provides an open line of access to all my past learning, to the experiences of my whole lifetime. It is rooted in an inner intuition and creativity that puts all this into a form which is useful in the here and now.

This is a meditative quality, a meditation in action, in life. Vipassana meditation offers us a model. It teaches an individual to be alert to and accepting of all that comes into consciousness, without repression or disturbance and without attachment. This means to actually acknowledge and accept what I feel or see, without trying to redirect, manage, or gloss over. Acceptance of what *is* opens the self to honesty, wonder, and appreciation. It teaches and requires love and respect for the life processes we all experience and witness.

My Body Is Physically Balanced

I move and work from my physical center, from my center of balance. This is important, both for my physical well-being as therapist, and as a living metaphor. When my body is not balanced, when my movements or position cause me stress, then I am coping with my stress. My stress communicates itself to every part of my body: back, neck, shoulders, arms, and hands. I am that much less open to what is occurring outside of me. And that stress is communicated to the client.

At times I am drawn to touch a specific place on the client's body. Then I realize that my position is uncomfortable. Is this a conflict between intuition and my well-being? No. At such times I gently and respectfully move back from the client and move my body. As I move physically I see or sense things differently. I usually realize that there is another, more comfortable way to do what intuition has suggested.

Some models of movement are helpful. Tai chi, Feldenkrais, or free-form dance can all help us to become more attuned to balance and flow in our movements so that we more naturally move in a way that is respectful of the body.

I Am Grounded

I repeatedly look to my feet, feel my feet as they provide my contact with the earth. Perhaps this is metaphorical, but it is a powerful physical metaphor for me. Standing, sitting, or moving, my feet are the foundation, the roots of my being. This awareness is a great help in maintaining physical and energetic balance.

I Keep Myself Energetically Open

I visualize my energy remaining free and clear, flowing to the earth and to the cosmos. Rather than think of protection in relation to the problems or pain of the client, I feel best thinking of freedom and flow in my own energy. As long as I have the inner resources to maintain this openness I feel invigorated and fascinated by the therapeutic process. When my own energy and resources are low I begin to become burdened by the therapeutic process, to feel constriction and pain in myself and in my life.

Then is the time to step back from being a therapist and take care of myself. This is as important as any skill, technique, or knowledge. As a therapist I am responsible for myself. If I am bringing pain to myself through the therapeutic process, then ultimately I am teaching the client to ignore self and endure pain.

The Circle of Learning

All of us have the capacity and the beginnings of these qualities. A wonderful thing about the therapy session is that these qualities can be called upon in a special way. For an hour or an hour and a half, I can maintain a focus, awareness, and openness that I am not capable of throughout the ordinary course of the day.

Experiencing the power of these qualities in the therapy session urges me to become more aware of their functioning in other aspects of my life. Being present, centered, and grounded becomes more widely available. Experimenting and bringing these qualities into play in my broader life enhances their effectiveness in the therapy session.

Release

One person needs only to touch another person's body with sensitivity, and it begins to respond to the energy of that touch. It softens and hardens, contracts and expands, moves sideways, lengthwise, or in an arc. Pain and pleasure can arise and dissipate. Breathing changes. Sounds from the belly herald a shifting of pressures and tensions around the digestive tract. Eyes describe patterns beneath the closed eyelids. Body parts may involuntarily jerk or shift.

All of these phenomena signal a shifting of inner energies in a process called *therapeutic release*. A focus of tension or rigidity is easing. Various fascias, ligaments, tendons, and muscle fibers, united in a pattern of strain or hypertonia, are finding a way to let go.

The signs of therapeutic release are so rich and varied because the total individual has been involved in a pattern of holding, the protective stiffness that the organism has used to cope with trauma. The nonconscious aspect of the person has accepted, even created this pattern. It involves capabilities of the immune system, of nerve, muscle, and connective tissue. It involves inner choice. To the conscious mind, the pattern of holding is most obvious as a chronic pain, a propensity to a specific injury, or a limitation of bodily function. It may also be reflected more subtly in posture, facial expression, sight, hearing, and freedom of choice. Thus the release of this pattern may involve muscle movement, sensations of pain, impressions of sight, sound, or posture, and indications that a person is momentarily in an altered state of consciousness.

For all the drama and allure of some of these manifestations, the physical patterns and changes seen and felt by the therapist are the surest guide through this searching and releasing. The words, emotions, and memories of the client are often very compelling, drawing both therapist and client to search into their meaning. Yet they may also be misleading, as our conscious expectations and curiosity guide us into paths that feel logical or powerful. The actual physical changes manifested by the client, the nonconscious tissue movements, provide a centering and grounding point in this process. Follow the tissue. Stay with the thought, the image, the words only as long as they are in harmony with the tissue change. Let go of words and movement when they stop naturally, or when they distract from the physical process. Let go of the whole process when there is a sense of completion.

Unwinding

An important part of therapeutic release is the searching of a body part through a pattern of movement. I use the word searching because that is what the body tissues appear to do. The motion may be circular, zigzag, or partially reverse itself. It may proceed rapidly, then return and go more slowly. To the therapist this pattern of movement often becomes the most obvious aspect of the release. Following and assisting this motion has come to be called *unwinding,* a basic and powerful technique of hands-on therapy. It is dealt with here because it is so fundamental to craniosacral therapy. Unwinding is a special aspect of therapeutic release that may come into play from the first moment of touch, or at the peak of a complex process of release.

The basis of unwinding is that the therapist moves with, supports, and moderates the nonconscious leading of the body tissue. Two examples of unwinding are the releases at the respiratory diaphragm and at the thoracic opening. There is no standard pattern of movement to look for or induce at those locations. The therapist follows, moving with what she feels in her hands.

In lending her energy, in moving with and continuing to follow the body, the therapist offers a type of support. The client's body accepts this as an opportunity to experiment with change, to explore the possibility of releasing self-imposed limitations. One step leads to the next in a sequence that is unpredictable to either client or therapist. The therapist offers reinforcement to this series of moves without getting ahead and without terminating abruptly.

The term *unwinding* especially applies to following and assisting the free movement of any body part at a joint. When the therapist is holding the client's head it may show a repeated tendency to turn off to one side. Carefully following this movement is a powerful way to assist in the release of the atlanto-occipital joint and the muscle and fascia connecting along the neck to the cranial base.

When working with the head or any other body part, it is important to offer full support, placing the hands so that there is very little weight on the joints or stress on the muscles.

It is also important to moderate the movement, to keep to a very gradual pace. Moving slowly, the tissue has time to release and to reorganize to indicate the next move. When the body part moves rapidly it appears to skip through a pattern that may have significance, but not to take time to release. If that happens the therapist can then follow through the pattern a second time, resisting rapid motion, while maintaining support and presence.

Practicing Unwinding

To practice unwinding, stand or sit to one side of your client. Let your posture be comfortable and relaxed. Gently grasp the client's arm, supporting it at elbow and wrist. Feel the energy of the arm. It may seem loose or tight, flexible or rigid. Do you sense a movement? Follow it very gradually, pausing as you go, alert for changes of direction. Be ready to move your body as necessary to keep centered and balanced, to offer full support to the arm.

The arm may move through a very wide range, or only very slightly. The benefit to the client has nothing to do with the amount of movement. A very small movement may result in profound relaxation in the arm and shoulder, or throughout the body.

You may practice unwinding at other parts of the body. Ankles, knees, or hips find release when we gently move the feet or legs. Always offer support and a gentle connection. Be aware of any area of contact between yourself and your client.

When the bones of the head appear to resist the directions traditionally prescribed for a release, they may find release through greater freedom of motion. Touch the sphenoid or frontal bone softly in the usual manner. Then, sit quietly, observing and offering no direction. When you notice a shifting, follow internally, support by your presence.

Unwinding, Range of Motion, and Micromovement

A special feel for range of motion is an important aspect of the unwinding we assist in craniosacral therapy. In massage, Shiatsu, or physical therapy, the therapist may move the arm or leg through a wide arc to test and extend range of motion. Often the therapist or client pushes directly against and through the body's resistance to achieve a greater range of movement. This produces the "pain that feels good." However, this is not the movement we use in craniosacral therapy. In my experience with unwinding, the client has no sense of stress because of the motion, but often a sense of wonder that such a range of motion feels so comfortable.

As you hold a body part, you support as much of the weight as possible. Center and ground yourself. Then follow any movement that seems to come from your hands or the client's body. Move very little and very slowly in one direction, hold, then take the movement in another direction. As you move, attend to resistance at a very subtle level. You may move less than a centimeter when you feel a slight hesitation or resistance in the muscles. If this happens, move in any other direction. The movement may be so slight that it is only a suggestion of a possibility. Be very responsive to any resistance, any reluctance. Move only in the direction, large or small, of greatest freedom—the direction of ease.

If the body part begins to move quickly, resist that movement enough to keep to a very slow pace. If you have been taken unawares and the body part has moved too quickly, allow the movement to complete. Then gently bring the body part back to the starting point, the place where rapid movement began. This time lightly resist the movement so that you maintain a gradual pace as you follow it. Often the greatest release occurs during this period when the therapist offers support, presence, and resistance to hurrying through.

This sensitivity is at the heart of craniosacral therapy.

Chapter 6

The Process of Assessment

Assessment in craniosacral therapy is a process of observation and unfolding experience. It is not completed by a careful judgment at the beginning of an encounter. Rather, assessment is a process that is alive throughout a session. As I move from place to place, I repeatedly open my awareness to indications which reach beyond my initial expectations. Through experience, I learn to attend to a wide range of signals emanating from the client and from my own inner sensations. These messages may be in the language of hard and soft tissue, of regular or irregular rhythms, of energy focus versus energy flow: they include all of the indications of release discussed in chapter 2.

Conventional medicine is based on a diagnosis; that diagnosis specifies the treatment. This is not helpful for craniosacral therapy, though the mind often yearns to encapsulate everything in a few words. Judgment and diagnosis have an air of finality about them. The more I think I know about this person, the less open I am to other possibilities. In reality, the processes and symptoms we observe are a small part of a broader pattern involving body, mind, and spirit. What is manifested to the mind and senses changes as we move through a therapeutic encounter. It is not necessary to know or plan everything in advance. Rather, we acknowledge and respond to the process moment to moment as it unfolds. Thus, assessment in craniosacral therapy is a process of uncovering, of discovery.

Impressions are formed, followed, and modified by immediate experience throughout the session.

The Client's Goal

The client usually approaches craniosacral therapy with a problem or a wish. At the beginning of a session, the therapist helps the client express what brings her here and what she hopes for. She may want to tell of pain or physical limitation. Beyond describing a problem, it is helpful for the client to express what she hopes for. The therapist can pose a few simple questions. Is there anything that you would like to tell me about your body? Do you have any difficulties you would like to describe? What do you hope for from this session? This last question is important for the client. It helps her to recognize and clarify her choices.

These questions are purposefully general. Listen and remember what your client has to say, but keep an open mind regarding the source of symptoms. We usually suppress many signals from the body in our eagerness to get on with daily life. The pain we feel is the aspect that reaches past our efforts at suppression. As a result, we usually are aware of only a part of the total picture.

Beginning the Session

At the beginning of a session, we form initial impressions. The listening stations provide an effective structure within which both client and therapist make contact. The therapist gains a general sense of the physical issues impacting the client. This gives a starting place for the work.

Simultaneously, the client is discovering manifold dimensions of the therapist. Qualities of touch, presence, and intent impress the client and begin to shape what will be revealed and explored within this duo.

As we move through the listening stations and begin the releases of the body, the pattern of energies and connections shifts. A curtain is parted and we are drawn to working in a way that would not have revealed itself at first. As points of pain or intense sensitivity are relieved, as balance returns within the body, so the overall pattern changes. As therapist, I wish to be awake and responsive to this shifting presentation.

The Value of Therapeutic Experience

At the beginning of our practice, we follow the treatment protocol presented in part 1. Repeated experience of these techniques enriches our learning. The hand positions become familiar. The touch becomes more natural as we get a feel for how it fits with a client's anatomy.

We recognize the craniosacral rhythm and its variations. We sense more accurately the resilience of joints and the quality of muscle and connective tissue throughout the body. Experience demonstrates to us the varied patterns of release across individuals. We witness the healing power of touch and support as we contact the body.

As we gain sensitivity through practice, we notice a growing sense of how and where to touch. At times, the hands seem to go to the exact point that will provide relief to the client, indicating some inner guidance system of which we are only vaguely aware. At other times, we feel an urge to move on, to change position. We discover that slight changes in hand position may greatly enhance the release process. Thus, we find that there are many more possibilities than the positions specified in the treatment protocol for each diaphragm.

The exercises and procedures in this chapter were developed in response to this type of experience. They are an attempt to understand and explain what happens as the therapist reaches beyond the box of traditional techniques and theories. Becoming more consciously aware of this natural process may help each therapist to become clearer about his or her perceptive capabilities. Our goal is that each individual discover how he or she most effectively tunes in, observes, and assists the client.

Modalities of Observation

We share the senses of sight, hearing, smell, and touch. As individuals we differ in the specific senses that convey the most meaning. We also differ in the way sense images illuminate our thinking. Some of us *see* an answer. Others *feel* the way. Though not exclusive, each modality helps an individual to observe and think effectively. Within the structure of therapy, each person's style brings greater life and effectiveness to her work. The following exercises are designed to explore how this style operates for you. The goal is to help each therapist become more consciously aware of the natural yet subtle ways she receives and uses information.

Looking

Standing a few feet away from the table, scan your client's body visually. Where are your eyes drawn? For many therapists this is the first step in assessment. This process may occur just below the level of consciousness: the therapist sees the client and immediately feels drawn to touch a particular place on the body.

We can develop this capacity when we do it consciously. Let your eyes scan softly. Keep them moving without pausing long to focus sharply. Where do the eyes want to go, where do they return: to one place, or more? This "looking" is not a process of judgment, nor is it specifically about posture. It is simply noting where the vision is drawn.

The goal is to go beyond the known and rational, to access the riches of our unconscious observation and communication. Thus, I may notice some obvious characteristics of posture or figure. My focus sharpens for a moment; I accept these points as my mind presents them. Then I consciously soften my vision and return to the global view that draws me, even if I do not comprehend its meaning.

Make a mental note of these observations before moving on to the other assessment modalities.

Sensing Physically

Standing close, as in the listening stations, I bring my energy inward, feeling my body and my connection with the ground. This helps the perception to broaden, to become general rather than sharply focused. Then, slowly moving one hand above the client, I let it come to rest on her body. I consciously let go of the positions and sequence dictated by the treatment protocol. I let the hand move freely, coming to rest where it is comfortable. After a few moments, I may do the same with the other hand. Rather than look intensely at this place, I look again to myself, to my center and ease of posture. This helps me to be broadly receptive to whatever may be communicated through touch and presence.

Do this as an exercise, opening to the unknown. What happens? Do you feel signs of release? How is it for your client? Remain open to sensory feedback: perhaps your hands will adjust position. Perhaps you will feel something specific about this location.

After a few minutes, lift one or both hands and notice if they seek a new position. Rather than thinking about it, just follow your hands. Let them rest awhile, and then move on. Have you experienced this before? What is the experience of your client?

Understanding Unconscious Perceptual Cues

The eye or the hand unconsciously seeks out a place on the body that is uncomfortable or constricted. This happens to many people, not only therapists. A silent communication occurs in nature. We observe that fish in a school or birds on the wing all turn together, with no obvious signal. How do we explain this? The mind searches for a key, some secret organ or scent that communicates along known scientific lines.

Going beyond the actual experience, therapists attempt to explain this perceptual phenomenon as follows.

When a part of the body experiences stress or injury, it responds protectively. Muscle tissue and fascia contract, thickening and stiffening. There is warmth, tightness, concentration of fluids, perhaps concentration of cellular waste products, a restriction of fluid and energy that would normally exchange more freely with surrounding tissue.

This type of restriction and congested energy may send out a signal that others can perceive below the level of conscious awareness. We find ourselves drawn intuitively by these signals to specific parts of the body, parts that are the locations of pain, tightness in connective tissue, and restriction of movement.

The signal is visualized as being transmitted in concentric circles, like ripples on a pond. Perhaps we sense these ripples, these arcs of energy, drawing us to the center, the point of discomfort. The term *arcing* has been used to describe this intuitive way of finding the part of the body that needs our attention.

This explanation is only a guess. However it is explained, both vision and touch can help us to perceive more broadly what the client is manifesting. The important thing is to recognize, develop, and use our inherent capabilities. We have capacities for perception, natural sensitivities, which lie dormant in modern technological society. We have been trained to disregard the messages from our bodies, to ignore intuition in order to cope with years of school and family. Yet, the body continues to offer to speak to each of us. People in more primitive societies respond naturally to subtle cues in nature and in one another. Often, life depends on their ability to recognize how their intuition works. We too can regain this ability, broadening our perceptual range.

Working with Symptoms

During the listening stations, my observations offer points for further investigation. As I sit to begin the releases, I may place my hand near one of these points to get a fuller sense of what is being communicated. As I touch, the tissue may begin to release. Or touching this point may lead me to other, connected places on the body. While I am in contact, the client may provide helpful feedback that did not occur to her when she was just thinking about the symptoms.

On the other hand, directly working at a symptomatic point is not always helpful. Touching may bring relief, or it may add a painful intensity in that area. Then it is more constructive to work around the intense areas, helping to restore flow to neighboring, seemingly empty and inactive tissue. This seems to bring strength and ease to surrounding tissue along with a dispersal of surplus energy from the painful region. It assists the whole body to achieve fuller flow and energetic balance.

I maintain this careful and open approach to the client throughout the session. At each release position, the body may offer feedback that helps me to modify my touch or opens my eyes to other possibilities. Sometimes I may move my hand slightly. At other times, one hand will stay in place while the other moves to a distant part of the body.

Throughout my work, I return my awareness to my body and posture. If my hand, arm, and body are comfortable, that is a clue that I am in the right place. If my hand is uncomfortable or wants to move, I shift it. As I move away from a conventional position, I often notice more signs of release in the client's body. Thus the nonverbal dialog between client and therapist offers many clues at each stage of the session.

Gentle Movement

This is another effective mode of presence and touch. Standing next to the massage table, touch the client's hip and softly rock it side to side. The amount of movement is very small, barely visible. Find the rhythm of the body by pushing lightly and following the return. Do not push against resistance. As the rocking motion starts, move with it, remaining in the barely perceptible range. Note the quality of the motion in the hips—is it free or constrained? Notice the way the movement is transferred upward to the chest and shoulders. Is it smooth or constricted? Notice the movement as it is transferred to the legs.

Move to the ribs and repeat this gentle rocking. Again, notice the quality of the movement in the chest and the quality of the connections above and below. Note the places where the motion is free, the places where it is constricted. As you discover something, the mind hones in and the view sharpens. Accept that, and return to a soft glance, to perceptual openness.

This motion is small, not disturbing, but gentle and comforting. It reveals characteristics of the joints, muscle, and connective tissue. We are able to see and feel areas of the body that are supple and free, and areas that are protectively constricted. This rocking technique may also be used on one leg at a time.

Experiment with using this assessment tool at any time during a session. As we gain experience, we gain a clearer view of the physical transitions from freedom to constriction. Moreover, the tissue often responds to this motion and begins to soften, the body to move more fluidly. Thus, it is a helpful adjunct to the more conventional forms of release.

This slight motion may also help the body to integrate the releases and energy shifts that have taken place during a session. You might find it interesting and useful to try it at the session's end.

Assessment as Dialog

Each person possesses a unique configuration of qualities, sensitivities, strengths, and weaknesses. These assessment procedures are a step in the process of reawakening and appreciating our inner capabilities. They offer us avenues for working with the reality of each client without preconceptions. They give a structure within which we learn to be receptive and open to new insights and new possibilities at every moment. Building on the structure of listening stations and releases, we learn to work in a way that is personal to each individual.

The process of assessment, of awareness, is interactive. The client, the body tissue, the physical organs respond to this particular person, this therapist, at this time and place. The dialog continues throughout the session: both client and therapist are learning to communicate effectively, to work together.

Evaluating the Craniosacral Rhythm

Because the craniosacral rhythm is a unique and central aspect of craniosacral therapy, a body of doctrine has grown up around it. Creative and innovative pioneers in the field have conjectured about what the rhythm is, what it means. Conjectures have later been taken as fact. Then more assumptions are made based on the previous ones. Many generalizations have been made about clients, based on the apparent rhythm.

Yet, we have not been able to measure this rhythm scientifically as an independent physiological phenomenon. Its basis is not clear. Moreover, the manner in which the rhythm manifests itself seems to vary, depending on the therapist.

Still, the rhythm manifests itself to thousands of therapists. The quality of the movements of the skeleton and cranium give cues to constriction and freedom within joints and tissue. In particular, the returning rhythm after a deep release process appears as a highly significant indicator of restored flexibility and freedom. Because I have experienced it, I accept the reality of a craniosacral rhythm. I recognize its cycle and its helpfulness in a session without knowing its physiological base.

If I must give a conventional scientific explanation for everything that I do, then I am confined by the concepts that I utilize. It is more realistic to be guided by the data of my experience, though I do not rationally understand exactly how they manifest themselves.

Layers of fascia form a supportive and protective structure around each organ and group of tissues in the body. Their protective constriction in the face of any trauma often restricts the natural motion of organs and joints in that area. Therapists observe that the motion of the craniosacral rhythm is also influenced. Thus, palpation of the rhythm has become a familiar assessment tool. Therapists have been monitoring this rhythm from the first days of their learning experience. Following is a review of the information we can gain from the craniosacral rhythm.

Symmetry

A difference from one side of the body to the other in the full cycle of the rhythm usually indicates a constriction of soft tissue above the point you are palpating. We think that the restriction is on the side that is slower, more ragged, or narrower in range of motion. Monitoring the rhythm at different places as you move up the body will help localize the problem.

Amplitude

The optimum rhythm is often felt after a release. The rhythm returns with a feeling of fullness, of wider spread and ease. A feeling of narrowness indicates constriction. It may be to one side only, resulting in an asymmetry as described above. Often a feeling of narrowness and constriction of the rhythm is felt on both sides together at one or two listening stations. And at times a sense of constriction in the rhythm appears very broadly through the body and the head.

When a sense of constriction extends over a broad section of the client's body, a specific focal point may not show up as the explanation. Usually, the muscles and connective tissue are also tight throughout the constricted region. Working carefully and attentively at the diaphragms usually results in a return of fullness in the rhythm and ease throughout the body.

Rate

The rate of the craniosacral rhythm may vary from four to twelve cycles a minute; it is usually slower than the rate of breathing at rest. Unlike the heart and breath, this rate usually does not vary from one situation to the next, when measured by the same therapist.

Different therapists may discover different rates of the rhythm. However, as therapists work together with the same client, the rhythms often come into synchrony. When a single therapist works with one client, the rhythms of therapist and client often move into synchrony.

Some leaders in the field have offered diagnostic conclusions based on the number of cycles each minute. These assumptions seem impressionistic. In my experience they are often not valid. Usually we find ourselves forming these judgments based on simple indicators when we do not understand a person well, or feel distant.

Quality

In addition to symmetry, amplitude, and rate, there may be another impression or quality conveyed by the rhythm. Pay attention to what you feel. You may sense struggle, peace, strength, withdrawal. Without putting too much emphasis on that impression alone, notice if it fits with other impressions and adds to your understanding of the client's experience.

A word of caution: The therapist's intuitive impression represents only one facet of the total being of the client. Intuition is often colored by a therapist's personal history. Be open to surprises and not too attached to any one sweeping view.

Working with the Dural Tube and the Spinal Column

The dural tube travels the length of the spine, furnishing a strong, protective, yet flexible outer sleeve for the environment of the spinal cord. It is continuous with the dural membrane of the cranial vault. But the dural tube only adheres to the spine at the upper cervical vertebrae and the sacrum. It is free through most of the spinal canal, able to adjust to body movement without constricting the nerve tissue of the spinal cord. At each vertebra, smaller sleeves emerge on each side of the dural tube, allowing nerve fiber to branch from the spinal cord to the body. These sleeves and their contents pass outward through spaces between the vertebrae, the intervertebral foramina.

At times, the dural tube may adhere to the side of the spinal canal, or become slightly twisted inside this space. This twisting may impede the flow of cerebrospinal fluid to parts of the spinal cord, or press on nerve trunks as they branch out from the cord to the body. To get a feeling for this, imagine the twisting that can occur along the sleeve of a jersey, or along the legs of tights. Remember the feeling of discomfort that can result by this slight torque pressure of fabric against skin.

Another type of restriction of the dural tube may be caused by misalignment. A misalignment between vertebrae may press against the dural tube, restricting movement and fluid flow. Usually a misalignment between vertebrae causes a pressure against one of the spinal nerves passing to the body. The result is pain and stiffness in the surrounding tissue. The gentle rocking mentioned previously helps relieve restrictions along the spine. In addition, the following visualization techniques can help you locate and relieve these restrictions.

Visualization and Flow

During the course of a session, you may be able to sense the quality of connection along the spine and the dural tube. This is especially true during the releases at the pelvis, at the atlanto-occipital joint, and at the parietal bones.

Palpation from the Sacrum or the Thoracic Opening

After performing the pelvic releases, let one hand remain in place at the sacrum. Let the fingers of the other hand touch the spinous processes of the lumbar spine. Move that hand step-by-step in either direction along the spine. Notice your impressions of freedom and restriction. Remain awhile, and feel the tissue softening, the communication opening along the spine.

You may also begin a similar process from the other end. Coming at an angle between shoulder and neck, gently place one hand behind the upper thoracic vertebrae as you did in the release of the thoracic diaphragm. Rest there a moment. Then, bring the fingers of the other hand to the spinal column around the respiratory diaphragm. Remain quietly in position as you observe changing signals from the body. Shift the hands as you feel inclined.

Palpation from the Occiput

After releasing the atlanto-occipital joint, relax your hands. Cradle the back of the head in your hands, with your fingertips lightly touching the base of the occiput. In your imagination, look down the dural tube. Visualize each vertebra. How far can you go? Do you sense freedom or restriction, comfort or discomfort? Do you feel a pulling on one side or the other? Test these impressions by comparing them to the client's report and to your feeling when you touch directly.

Palpation from the Parietal Bones

As the parietal release completes, sit quietly with your fingers in place on the parietals. With your inner perception, "look" through the falx cerebri, across the tentorium cerebelli to the dura mater as it passes through the foramen magnum to form the dural tube. You may sense restriction or openness in any of these membranes. Do you feel any influence from the musculature of the shoulders?

Synchronization at Occiput and Sacrum: Bridging

The craniosacral rhythm is characterized by recurring movement in all the bones and tissues of the cranium and the spinal column. Unless there is some disturbing influence, the occiput and the sacrum move in unison through the cycle. As the occiput rotates out and downward toward the feet, the spine seems to lengthen. The sacrum rotates so that the tip of the sacrum (the coccyx) rocks forward (to the anterior). As the occiput rotates inward and upward, the spine seems to shorten, and the tip of the sacrum rocks back (to the posterior).

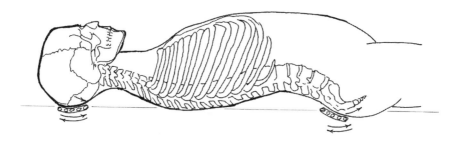

Figure 50. Bridging Occiput and Sacrum. Rhythmic pressure changes throughout the cranial vault and spinal canal produce a similar rocking motion in the occiput and the sacrum: downward on flexion, upward on extension. Arrows on the occiput and at the sacrum indicate the motion of flexion. This motion can be palpated and enhanced by placing your hands behind these points as the client is lying on a padded table. Double sets of arrows indicate the motion perceived by the therapist's hands.

This motion can be palpated at almost anytime during the session. To get a feeling for this motion, hold your hands forward in front of you, palms up and slightly cupped. Then rotate each of them in a small arc, moving from the wrist. The hands move together, both tilting to one side, then to the other. Elbows and forearms are relatively still, merely accommodating to the motion of hands and wrists. This is merely a suggestion of the subtle movements we feel on the body.

To palpate this movement on your client, sit to one side, facing the massage table. Reaching in from the side, contact the sacrum with the fingers of one hand. Place the other hand under the back of the head, cradling the occiput. Ensure that both you and your client are comfortable.

Let your arms relax. Observe any motions or signals of release at either hand. As the motion of sacrum and occiput become clearer to you, notice how closely they move in unison. If the motion is synchronized, the hands will seem to move or rock together. You may notice differences in the strength of movement between occiput and sacrum.

In its traditional form, this release specifies that you exert a slight pressure emphasizing the motion at each end of the spine. This is in effect a traction of the spine and the dural tube. By your presence and slight emphasis, you may assist in bringing occiput and sacrum into harmony, both in timing and in amplitude of movement. If you notice restrictions, look inwardly along the dural tube for their source. Be aware that your hands may be imposing restrictions if they are uncomfortable to you or to your client.

You can also practice bridging between regions on the spine and body. Starting with one hand as the anchor, we contact points along the spine with the fingertips of the other hand. Touching in this way is physically more comfortable than holding the head and the sacrum at the same time. Working in smaller steps, we help the body reestablish communication and ease among its parts. We touch lightly, allowing time for release, softening, and integration at each step. The body itself does the work.

At times, I begin with my hands near one another, as in the release of the lumbosacral joint. Then I move one hand up the spine. At other times, it seems more effective to begin with a greater span and move closer in steps.

There is no rule, except to remain open and respectful of the client and of the therapeutic relationship.

Using These Assessment Procedures in a Session

These procedures provide a variety of methods of tuning in or discovering what the client's body is willing to reveal here and now. Practicing these techniques can help to deepen your awareness of the subtle modes the body can use to signal its status. At first it may be helpful to experiment with all of these techniques, getting a feel for each one. Use them with the listening stations or mix them in during the diaphragm releases. With experience you will discover which feels most comfortable, which fits best with your individual skills.

Most of these procedures give indications of energy intensity, of energy blockage. It is interesting to note patterns. Do focal points cross from side to side? For example, the right hip may feel painful or restricted, and the left upper abdomen around the stomach or the spleen. Or does restriction appear to hold to one side? For instance, the shoulder, the ribs, and the hip may all feel restricted on the same side. Some therapists mark the results of their initial evaluation on a chart of the human body. They can then refer to it from session to session and note changes. Besides a useful record-keeping technique, this can be a helpful learning tool.

Chapter 7

The Cranial Vault

This chapter is presented as a review and an expansion on what you already know about the cranial vault. The information presented goes beyond what is essential to work effectively as a craniosacral therapist. However, it may answer some questions, and stimulate others. In particular I hope that the feel for the cranial vault communicated here will deepen your appreciation and wonder at the life processes we briefly contact and assist.

A Special Environment

The cranial vault and the spinal canal comprise a unique and specialized environment within the human organism. The notion of *vault* implies protection and safety. These are provided by the bony framework, by successive layers of membrane, and by a fluid bath that surrounds the entire central nervous system.

A structure that is merely strong may be made vulnerable by its rigidity. Flexibility and resilience are also of crucial importance. These qualities are provided by the joints and tissues connecting the bones, and by the quality of the bones themselves. This combination of strength and resilience varies from the top of the skull to its base, and from the fine bones of the neck to the heavy structures of the lowest vertebrae and the sacrum. All have the capacity to absorb and dampen shock, to respond to changes in internal or external pressure, and to recover from shock or stress.

Finally, the health and effective functioning of the central nervous system requires free flow into and out of the cranial vault and the spinal canal. Special openings at the base of the cranial vault and along the length of the spinal column provide for the passage of fluid and nerve impulse in both directions.

A Detailed Look at the Cranial Vault

We will now consider the construction and functioning of the cranial vault in greater detail. In the environment of the cranial vault, fluid, membrane, and bones interact to establish a place of protection, nurturing, and effective activity. An understanding of the interactive functioning of this environment gives us a greater awareness of our role as therapists. We touch this system from outside, assisting its return to harmony.

Brain and Nerve Tissue

The vault encloses the brain, a special center for receiving, processing, and distributing information. Messages pass to and from the cells of the

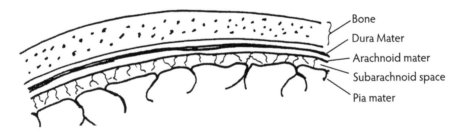

Figure 51. Membrane Layers of the Cranial Vault. The arachnoid membrane is backed by the dura and sends filaments through the subarachnoid space to the pia mater. The pia mater adheres to the brain surface, following all its folds. Cerebrospinal fluid flows within the subarachnoid space.

brain to every part of the body. The cranial nerves and the spinal nerves provide avenues of communication between the total organism and the processing or thought centers of the central nervous system.

Fluids

Nerves are not the only pathways between the brain and the body. Messages also pass by way of the fluids entering and leaving the cranial vault. Arteries and veins pass through openings (foramina) in the floor of the cranial vault. The flow of blood contributes to the pressure balance within the vault and provides life-sustaining fluid, nourishment, and protective cells. Electrolyte and hormone levels in the blood send signals to the brain about the body and its organs.

Within the cranial vault the pineal and pituitary glands are intimately connected with brain tissue. These glands release hormones into the bloodstream, sending their own messages from the cranial vault to glands, organs, and individual cells throughout the body. A free flow of nerve impulse and fluid in and out of the vault are clearly as important to the whole organism as is the physical integrity of the vault's outer shell.

Fluid and Membranes

The brain and spinal cord are immersed in a fluid that is produced and absorbed within the protective environment of the meninges, the membranes between brain and bone. The cerebrospinal fluid is something like lymph in consistency. Yet it flows chiefly within its own system. Produced within spaces in the brain's center and stem, it flows around the brain and spinal cord and is absorbed again into the bloodstream near the brain's upper surface.

Fluid and membrane are partners in forming the protective, nourishing environment around the brain. A tough outer membrane, the dura mater, is chiefly concerned with establishing the integrity of the outer shell. It is so closely bonded to the periosteum of the bones that it is almost indistinguishable from it. The dura mater also folds inward to form the falx cerebri, the falx cerebelli, and the tentorium cerebelli. These partitions provide increased stability to the brain mass by building partitions between its major parts.

The delicate innermost membrane, the pia mater, adheres directly to the surface tissue of the brain and spinal cord, following all its folds and lining all its cavities. Between the pia mater and the dura mater is the arachnoid mater. Backed by the dura, it sends thin filaments inward, forming bridges to its neighbor, the pia mater. This forms the subarachnoid space. Here, between the arachnoid and pia membranes, is the environment of the cerebrospinal fluid.

Within the brain itself, near each side and in the center, are hollows, known as ventricles. The pia mater, following all the folds and channels of brain tissue, lines these inner spaces. Within the ventricles, blood capillaries swell up from the surface of the pia mater. The capillaries gather into clumps, which secrete cerebrospinal fluid. This cluster is called the choroid plexus.

Cerebrospinal fluid fills the two lateral ventricles and flows into the third, central ventricle, increasing in volume. It then passes through the cerebral aqueduct of the brain stem into the fourth ventricle. From there, openings allow cerebrospinal fluid to enter and flow within the subarachnoid space. Cerebrospinal fluid also flows directly from the fourth

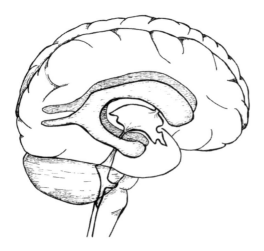

Figure 52. The Ventricles. These four fluid-filled hollow spaces deep within the brain are the chief sources of cerebrospinal fluid for the central nervous system. The two lateral ventricles lie within the left and right hemispheres of the brain. Their fluid secretions pass into the irregularly shaped third ventricle and then to the fourth ventricle in the brain stem. Cerebrospinal fluid passes from here into the central canal of the spinal cord and into the subarachnoid space around the brain and the spinal cord.

ventricle into the central canal of the spinal cord. It circulates down the central canal and the back of the spinal cord and up the front of the spinal cord.

Cerebrospinal fluid continually circulates within all the spaces around the brain and spinal cord. During its passage, some of the fluid seeps away from the central nervous system into intracellular tissues. Here it blends with interstitial fluid to be carried away by the lymph system. Much of the fluid continues within its specialized environment until it is absorbed at the arachnoid granulations.

Near the top of the head, portions of the arachnoid membrane penetrate the walls of the large vessels, which carry venous blood. These penetrations are called the arachnoid villi. As they expand with age to form small chambers, they become known as the arachnoid granulations. Here cerebrospinal fluid is drawn out of the subarachnoid space to be absorbed into the venous bloodstream.

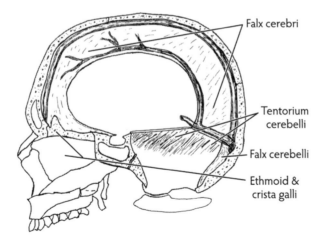

Figure 53. The Falx and the Tentorium. Layers of the dura mater fold inward to form protective compartments within the cranial vault. The sickle-shaped falx forms a central partition between the hemispheres of the cerebrum and the cerebellum. The tentorium spreads protectively to each side over the cerebellum. The falx cerebri and tentorium cerebelli also support large channels for the return of venous blood. Illustrated above are the superior and inferior sagittal sinuses, embedded in the falx cerebri, and the connecting straight sinus.

There is a thin flow of cerebrospinal fluid around the entire brain and spinal cord. In addition, small reservoirs of fluid collect in the uneven spaces between nerve tissue and outer membrane. These occur around the fourth ventricle, at the base of the brain, and at the sacrum. Thus, the brain and spinal cord are surrounded, almost floating in cerebrospinal fluid.

Fluid and layers of membrane cushion the brain and spinal cord. As cerebrospinal fluid flows over the pia mater of brain and cord, it provides both nourishment and waste removal. It ensures the proper balance of electrolytes and circulates specialized immune bodies between the meninges.

The Cranial Rhythm

Since the time of William Sutherland, therapists have been aware of a regular cyclic movement separate from breathing and heartbeat. It can be felt on the bones of the head and spine as the craniosacral rhythm, or the cranial rhythmic impulse. Somehow, this motion is reflected throughout the body, so that a component of the craniosacral rhythm can be felt in the feet, the legs, the pelvis, and the ribs. Its effect on the bones of the head will be discussed more fully in the next two chapters.

Sutherland and others have attributed this movement to cycles in the production and absorption of cerebrospinal fluid. Unfortunately, this has never been verified outside the circles of craniosacral therapy. The pressure changes and movements seem to be too subtle to be measured by instruments in common use.

The Bones of the Cranial Vault

The bones of the cranial vault vary tremendously depending on their location and function, but all contribute to a container possessing strength, light weight, and flexibility. Near the top of the head, the bony surfaces that provide outward protection are smooth and simple. Their gently curved forms build a strong and compact inner space. The parietal bones most directly represent this outer, visible structure.

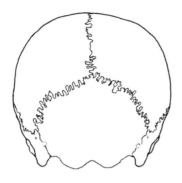

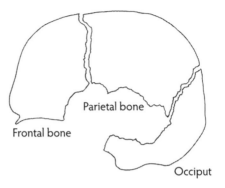

Parietal bone

Frontal bone

Occiput

Figure 54a. The Interlocking Sutures of the Cranial Vault. These secure joints have the capability of adapting to stress or pressure changes.

Figure 54b. A Diagrammatic Left-side View. The frontal bone and the occiput curve under to form a part of the cranial base. The parietal is the only bone of the vault that does not reach into the base.

Unlike the upper skull, where the bones join in long, curving sutures, the joints of the cranial base form jagged and abruptly turning lines. The central portion of the cranial base is made up of several thick but narrow sections, giving both strength and flexibility. This structure has the capacity to dampen, absorb, and adapt to the changing stresses, jolts, and pressures which come upward from the torso or are telegraphed directly along the spinal column.

Flexibility is achieved partially by the bone matter itself. The bones are not rigid like a dried wood, but flexible, like a living tree. They can give a little without cracking.

Rather than form a single shell, the cranial vault is composed of many curved plates joined by interlocking seams known as sutures. This type of joint grips tightly yet allows for slight movement. The effect of a suture can be imagined to be like the effect of joining hands by interweaving the fingers. The fingers provide a secure connection where they meet, yet allow movement of the hands and wrists. The container formed by this type of joint can flex and shift in response to inner or outer pressure. The interwoven fingers of bone are clothed in the periosteum. This connective tissue provides an added cushion and flexibility at the sutures. The dura mater, the inner connective tissue in which the bones are embedded, adds resilience. The dura gives shape to the container. It holds the bones in position and attempts to return them to their original position when distortion has occurred.

On the other hand, the dura mater may protectively tighten as a response to stress or trauma. Then it gives up some of its resilience in order to hold the bones tightly together at their sutures. It is the connective tissues, the dura and the periosteum, which respond to touch. To speak metaphorically: sensing the supportive presence of the therapist's hands, these tissues are able to let go their extreme vigilance. Relaxing their level of tension, they sort through other possibilities. They are searching for a more comfortable level of holding with resilience. This level of renewed ease is not some standard formula that applies to everyone. A unique combination of energy, vigilance, and ease will be effective for each different person.

The Frontal Bone

The frontal, the bone that faces forward to the world, is one of the most solid structures of the head. It curves from the coronal suture forward, slopes downward to form the forehead, and then turns back in above the eyes. This wraparound, curved structure gives great strength to the forehead. A narrow slit in its floor allows the ethmoid bone access to the vault. Otherwise, the frontal bone completely encloses the forepart of the brain on all sides. Its shape resembles a half sphere, flattened and molded across its base.

The coronal suture, where the frontal joins the two parietal bones, is relatively simple. As the posterior edge of the frontal curves down on each side, it meets the greater wing of the sphenoid. The wings and body of the sphenoid then form an extensive joint with the lower edge of the frontal, behind the eyes. The sphenoid and frontal bones flatten to form a broad, rough triangle where they join at the outer corner of each eye. The frontal seems to rest on the sphenoid here. Directly inside the sphenoid, medially from this heavy joint, are passages for nerves and blood vessels to

Figure 55a. The Frontal Bone from Inside. This sagittal section depicts the sutures of the frontal bone with the parietal bone and the greater wing of the sphenoid. Beginning at the coronal suture, the frontal curves forward to the hairline, downward at the forehead, and back above the eyes to meet the sphenoid.

Directly behind the bridge of the nose a narrow slit in the frontal bone allows the ethmoid bone (not pictured here) to reach into the vault. The sphenoid and its wings reach across the width of the skull, joining the lower edge of the frontal behind and on the outer side of each eye. (See also figures 58a and 58b.)

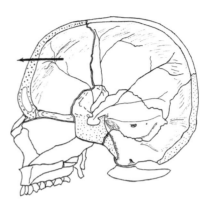

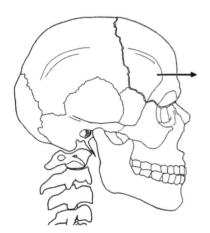

Figure 55b. An Outside View of the Frontal Bone. Beyond the cranial vault, the bones of the nose, mouth, and face join the frontal. The direction of release is traditionally considered to be forward, away from the parietal and sphenoid bones. At times, the bones around the orbit, nose, and face may be felt to be providing some resistance to the release. As you follow the frontal release, the movement may feel irregular or vary from side to side as restrictions in the dura mater gradually release along the sutures.

the eyes and face. An outer flange of bone protects this joint. The zygoma stretches downward from the frontal, across the edge of the sphenoid, to the surface of the maxilla.

The base of the frontal bone reaches back above each eye, forming a curved roof for the eye socket. Between the eyes, above the inner passages of the nose, the ethmoid, lacrimal, maxillary, and nasal bones join the frontal. Please refer to figures 73 and 83 in chapter 9.

Because of these complex connections, the connective tissue may hold the frontal bone more firmly across its base than it does along the coronal suture. The motion of the frontal seems to be especially influenced by the motion of the sphenoid. The extensive joints along its lower edge and at each temple draw the frontal in the direction of the sphenoid.

The ideal direction of release is thought to be directly forward from the face. Restriction most often appears somewhere along the base of the frontal bone, around the eyes. What I look for in working with the frontal is not release in a specific direction, but a greater ease and range in its movement.

The Ethmoid

The ethmoid is the one bone of the cranial vault that we do not directly contact in palpating the skull. Nestled between the eyes, it is directly below the center of the frontal bone. Much of the ethmoid forms the nasal passages and houses the sense of smell.

The construction of the ethmoid is unusual. Air cells with thin, bony walls form labyrinthine chambers on each side of a perpendicular plate. This fragile structure extends from the maxilla and lacrimal bones at the bridge of the nose back to the sphenoid and palatine bones. Each side of the ethmoid forms the inner wall of each eye socket. The lower folds of these chambers roof the nasal passages on each side.

The ethmoid's central, perpendicular plate contributes to the nasal partition, the septum. Its lower edge joins another thin partition, the vomer. Reaching upward beyond the body of the ethmoid, its perpendicular plate passes into the cranial vault through a narrow slit in the floor of the frontal bone. Here, this extension of the ethmoid forms a special anchoring point, the crista galli, for the falx cerebri. (See figure 53.)

Within the frontal slit, a denser bone known as the cribriform plate forms the roof of the ethmoid. Tiny openings allow passage for blood vessels and nerves from the cranial vault into the chambers of the ethmoid. (See figures 60 and 61.) The inner portions of these chambers are shaped into contours that swirl the air over the mucous membrane and hair follicles of the nasal passages. Sense receptors for smell are here, directly beneath the frontal lobes of the brain.

Figure 56a. The Parietal Bones: An Inside View.
Both views depict the sutures of the parietal bone
with the frontal, sphenoid, temporal, and occipital
bones. (Not shown is the sagittal suture along the
top between the parietal bones.)

The coronal suture between the parietal and
frontal bones curves down to the temple on each
side. Here the parietal briefly meets the sphenoid,
then follows back along the irregular curve of the
temporal bone.

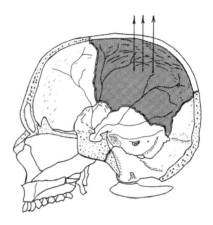

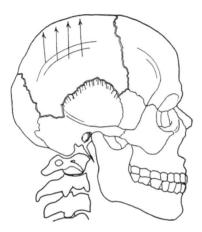

Figure 56b. The Parietal Bones from the Outside. The
squamous suture between the temporal and parietal
bones is beveled, so that the temporal bone slightly
overlaps the parietal on each side (indicated by slashes).
At the occiput, the parietal bone follows the lambdoid
suture diagonally upward toward lambda, just above the
external occipital protuberance. The traditional direction
of release is upward, as illustrated by the arrows.

Though we do not feel the motion of the ethmoid directly, we probably affect its sutures as we work with the frontal, the sphenoid, and later
the vomer, maxillas, and nasal bones. We will return to the ethmoid in
chapter 9.

The Parietal Bones

The parietals exemplify the smooth, simple structure of the bones forming the outer surface of the cranial vault. They are the only bones that
do not also fold inward to form part of the cranial base. The two parietal
bones join at the sagittal suture, which extends along the center of the

skull from the frontal bone to lambda, the point where the parietal bones meet the occiput.

Within the cranial vault, below the sagittal suture, the dura mater forms the falx cerebri, a partition between the hemispheres of the brain. This is the partition of connective tissue that extends from the ethmoid and frontal bones to the occipital protuberance. Folded into the falx, along its length, is a large venous blood vessel, the superior sagittal sinus. (See figure 53.) It is into this space that the arachnoid granulations press, to return cerebrospinal fluid to the bloodstream.

The filling phase of the craniosacral rhythm presses the parietal bones outward and upward. As we assist in their release by drawing upward, we contact the falx, releasing accumulated stress in this inner structure of the dura mater. Through the falx, the release may extend downward, into the tissues of the cranial base and the neck.

Most of the lower side of the parietal bone is beveled where it is overlapped by the temporal bone along the squamous suture. The overlapping temporal produces a cup effect, holding the lower edges of the parietal bones.

The Temporal Bones

At each side of the head, the simplicity of the parietal bones gives way to the multifunctional temporal bones. Each temporal bone is relatively flat in a semicircular section above and around the ear. The upper edge of the bone is beveled where it overlaps the parietal bone. The temporal bone becomes irregular in shape along its lower edge. It thickens and narrows as it reaches inward between the sphenoid and the occiput. This heavier section is host to a variety of functions.

Along the lower edge of the temporal bone, the zygomatic process reaches forward, a hollowed space presents a joint for the lower jaw, the ear canal slopes inward, and the mastoid process develops as an important point of tissue attachment.

Just in front of the ear canal, the lower jaw forms a sliding hinge with the temporal bone. Slightly above that joint, an extension of the temporal arches forward to the zygoma. The muscles of mastication reach upward

Figure 57a. The Temporal Bones: An Inside View.
In these flattened drawings the temporal bones are
at center on each side. The drawing at right looks
downward into the inside of the cranial base. The
drawing below looks upward at the outer features of
the base. The arrows originating at the outer ear canal
indicate approximately the traditional direction of
release. Note that this conforms roughly to the angle
of the petrous portion in the base. The direction of
release is traditionally considered to be diagonally
outward and backward.

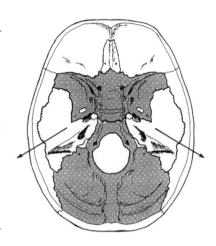

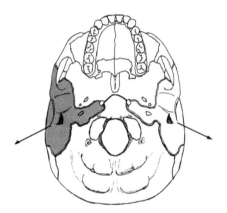

Figure 57b. The View from Below. Even in this
seemingly straightforward release, it is important to
follow the motion of the bones, as they reflect the
stress patterns and softening of the dura mater along
the sutures. Release of the temporal bones can make
a great contribution to the release of the cranial base,
including restrictions in the dura mater around the
foramina at the edges of the temporal bone.

from the mandible, flowing beneath the zygomatic arch. They attach in a
wide arc along each side of the skull. Thus, movements of the jaw directly
affect the temporal, parietal, sphenoid, and frontal bones.

Behind the ear is the rounded knob known as the mastoid process. It
provides an attachment for neck muscle that reaches upward from breastbone and clavicle. Muscles also reach forward from the mastoid process
into the floor of the mouth. Nearby, the styloid process projects downward.
It provides additional attachment for ligament and muscle to the hyoid
bone and the tongue or floor of the mouth.

At times people experience tightness or pain in the muscles of the jaw and at the temporomandibular joint. Usually this constriction radiates upward from the neck and shoulders and influences muscles and connective tissue all around the neck and cranial base. Therefore, relaxing the upper torso, the shoulders, the neck, and the cranial base is an important preliminary to bringing relief to the jaw and its muscles.

The underside of the temporal bone narrows into an inward projection, the petrous part. It reaches like a finger into the cranial base, up to the joint between the occiput and the sphenoid. Its thickness forms a solid case for the delicate mechanisms of hearing and the sense of equilibrium. Inside the vault, the petrous portion of the temporal bone serves as an anchor for the tentorium cerebelli, a partition of dural membrane over the cerebellum. When there is constriction of the cranial base, release of the connective tissue and joints of the temporal bone is as important as release of the sphenoid and occiput.

The Occiput

In contrast to the sturdy frontal bone, the occiput, the bone at the back of the head, is so thin that it flexes outward and inward with the pulse of the craniosacral rhythm. On the inside it is marked by ridges that cross each other. These ridges provide attachment for the falx cerebri, the falx cerebelli, and the tentorium cerebelli. The meeting of these inner partitions of the vault is marked outwardly by the external occipital protuberance. An external ridge falling in a gentle arc toward the mastoid process marks the inner attachment of the tentorium cerebelli and provides outer muscle attachment.

Muscles of the neck extend downward from their lines of attachment across the outer surface of the occiput. These muscles and dense layers of fascia form a heavy curtain of rearward protection for the upper cervical vertebrae and their junction with the occiput.

The bone of the occiput thickens and becomes narrower as it curves down and inward to make up its portion of the cranial base. Around the foramen magnum the bone forms a smooth lip over which the dural membrane passes as it enters the spinal column.

The atlanto-occipital joints are on either side of the foramen magnum. Two smooth, rounded surfaces are formed: the occipital condyles. These rest on the upward-facing facets of the atlas, the slender first vertebra. The condyles are portrayed on the outer illustration for the temporal bones. (See figure 57b.) The position of the atlas is represented in the sphenoid illustration (figure 58b). These joints allow a rocking motion of the head, as in nodding yes. Constriction of the muscles reaching upward from the back and neck may compress and limit the motion at this joint. A habitual tightening of the muscles that reach the occiput may induce a protective tightening at the sutures all around the occiput. As we work upward from the torso, we assist the relaxation of the tissue of the upper body, the shoulders, and the neck. The atlanto-occipital release induces a softening of the dense connective tissue and muscle around this joint. Less constriction in the supporting tissue allows freedom and mobility at the joint and in the connective tissue all around the occiput.

Extending beyond the foramen magnum, the basilar part of the occiput narrows more and sweeps upward, establishing a strong angular reinforcement above the occipital condyles. Here it meets the body of the sphenoid at the sphenobasilar synchondrosis. (See figure 58a.) In this special joint, a thin pad of cartilage between the bones allows a limited hinging action.

A narrow finger of the temporal bone reaches inward on each side of the joint between the sphenoid and the occiput, forming a buffer or gasket between the wider portions of the occiput and the sphenoid. Thus the vault's floor is strongly reinforced to carry the weight of the entire head, yet it is composed of many segments, providing both flexibility and the ability to absorb impact and stress. The multiple segments of the cranial base might be compared to the interconnected boards of a footbridge suspended from cables. This loose construction from many parts provides a solid footing, yet allows supple movement among the parts.

The Sphenoid

The sphenoid is nestled in the middle of the cranial base. It shares a suture with every other bone in the cranial vault. Thus, its motion reflects the freedom or constriction of every other part of the cranial vault. The body

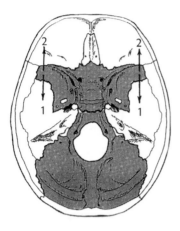

Figure 58a. The Sphenoid in the Cranial Base.

The sphenoid is central to the cranial base and touches every other bone in the cranial vault. In the view to the left, both the sphenoid and the occiput are shaded. Below, only the body and wings of the sphenoid are shaded.

The rhythmic motions of the sphenoid and the occiput are complementary. As shown below, the occipital condyles rest on the facets of the atlas, which act as a fulcrum. This gives the occiput a levering action as it moves over the atlas. The thin cartilage pad at the joint between the sphenoid and the occiput allows a hinging motion. As each bone rocks down and away from the center of the vault, their joint is pushed upward slightly by the base of the occiput. The curved arrows below indicate this motion. It can be palpated at the back of the head and at the temples.

Release of restrictions in the dura mater along the sutures is traditionally accomplished through movement in two directions. Numbered arrows indicate the sequence of these movements.

First, compression. The sphenoid is followed in a posterior direction. This compresses its sutures with the occiput and with the petrous portion of the temporal bone. This direction of movement also provides space at the sphenoidal sutures with the frontal and the ethmoid bones.

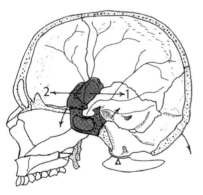

Figure 58b. A Side View.

Second, decompression. The sphenoid is followed in an anterior direction, providing space at its sutures with the occiput and the temporal bones and compressing its sutures with the frontal and the ethmoid bones.

These two motions exercise the dura mater along all of the sutures of the sphenoid. With the release of restrictions there is a return of flexibility and a broader range of movement among the bones of the cranial base. This release also allows the relaxation of the sleeves of dura mater around the nerves and blood vessels passing through the walls of the cranial vault.

of the sphenoid forms a narrow and strong bridge across the floor of the cranial vault. Within the sphenoid's thick central body, the sella turcica provides a specially protected pocket for the body's master gland, the pituitary. This central portion arches over the posterior nasal passages, above the open passageway of the throat. (See figure 58b.)

To each side, the wings of the sphenoid flare outward and upward, giving it the shape of a butterfly. These wings lie inward from the temples. We palpate them on each side above the zygomatic arch, just behind the corner of the eye. The greater wings of the sphenoid reach between a convergence of the frontal, the parietal, and the temporal bones. The feet of the butterfly, the sphenoid's pterygoid processes, reach directly downward around the nasal septum. They provide anchors for muscles of the jaw and support the palatine bones.

Across its front edge, behind and above the eyes, the sphenoid forms an extensive joint with the frontal bone. A central slit interrupts this wide joint, where the ethmoid thrusts through the frontal to anchor the falx cerebrum. The ethmoid joins the sphenoid behind the bridge of the nose. It forms the center and folds of the nasal passages, and links to the vomer, which also connects to the lower center of the sphenoid. Thus the bony structure of the nose is intimately connected to the cranial vault, particularly the sphenoid. This structure reflects the motions and constrictions of the cranial bones and communicates them to the maxillas.

Together the sphenoid and frontal bones form much of the orbit of the eye. Many branches of the cranial nerves pass directly through foramina in the sphenoid to muscles and sense receptors of the eyes, mouth, face, and teeth. Constriction in the tissues around the nerves may result in pain or limited function anywhere in this area. The solution is usually very simple. The procedures of the full protocol, with the addition of simple attention to the bones of the mouth and face, bring release through the whole area. This usually restores normal movement as well as nerve and fluid flow.

The Motions of Sphenoid and Occiput

The rhythmic motions of sphenoid and occiput are complementary. During the phase of flexion, or outward motion, the broader portions of both bones move downward, away from the center of the vault. However, the motion of the occiput is restricted by its connection to the atlas, which acts as a fulcrum. As the broader, posterior part of the occiput moves outward, it rocks on the atlas, causing the occiput's narrow base to tilt upward toward center. The base of the occiput carries with it the base of the sphenoid. As the body and wings of the sphenoid move downward, its narrow base is constrained and tilted upward with the occiput. Thus, both sphenoid and occiput move in a rocking action that is allowed by their special connection, the sphenobasilar synchondrosis.

William Sutherland, focusing on the changes of angle between sphenoid and occiput at their joint, called these movements *flexion* and *extension*. Following Sutherland's terminology, these words have come to be associated with any body movement related to the cycle of the craniosacral rhythm.

Chapter 8

Releasing the Cranial Base

The cranial base is the floor of the cranial vault. Parts of the frontal, sphenoid, temporal, and occipital bones form this floor. The ethmoid makes a small but significant contribution where it reaches through a notch in the floor of the frontal bone. In contrast to the smoothness and relative simplicity of the bones and joints on the top and sides, the base of the skull is uneven and complex. The sutures are close to one another and follow irregular lines, giving greater flexibility. Many openings allow the passage of nerves and fluid. Hollows provide space for the pituitary gland and for the organs of sight, smell, and hearing. Projections and knobs provide a base for the bones of the face and allow the attachment of muscle and ligament that reach to the jaw, the neck, and the shoulders.

The sphenoid is the central bone in this structure. It has special significance because it touches every other bone in the cranial vault. Thus, constriction of the connective tissue between bones and variations of movement in any of the bones of the cranium interact with the movement of the sphenoid. Moreover, the sphenoid, frontal, and temporal bones support and interact with the bones of the mouth and the face.

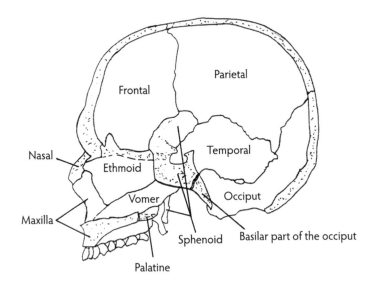

Figure 59. The Bones of the Cranial Vault,
the Face, and the Mouth.
A mid-sagittal section.

The normal condition of cranial bones, dura mater, and other connective tissue involves almost continuous rhythmical and harmonious movement. Probably this is the natural condition of all body tissues and organs. In addition to the rhythmic movement of structures, there is a continuous flow of communication, fluid, and energy among all parts of the head and body.

As with other structures of the body and head, our hands contact the bones of the cranial base. The quality and direction of their movement conveys information. We receive cues regarding the condition of the connective tissue around and between the cranial bones, especially the dura mater.

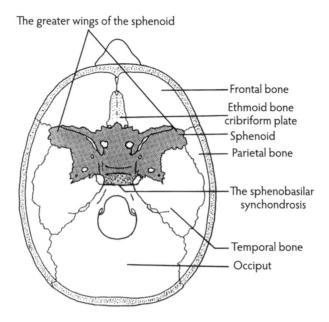

The greater wings of the sphenoid

Frontal bone
Ethmoid bone
cribriform plate
Sphenoid
Parietal bone
The sphenobasilar
synchondrosis
Temporal bone
Occiput

Figure 60. A View of the Cranial Base. Looking downward, into the cranial vault.

As our hands move from place to place on the head, we sense patterns of movement within the structure as a whole. These patterns may indicate areas of constriction in the connective tissue within the skull. Moreover, as we touch, we may sense a relationship to holding patterns below in the neck, the shoulders, and the torso.

Ideally, all of these parts move in harmony; there is a balance from side to side. Yet, when a tissue or organ is restricted in movement, then other parts adapt, establishing a new "harmony" that balances and compensates, but that may result in irregularities of flow and function. The original constriction may be a protective response to physiological stress or to injury. Or it could result from prolonged life stress. Eventually, all parts of the body become involved in the adaptation. For instance, imbalances in the sacrum or pelvis are reflected downward to the knees and ankles and upward to the shoulders and cranial bones. Tight shoulders may eventually extend down to the lower back and up to the neck, jaw, and cranial base.

Within the cranial vault, localized restrictions in the periosteum and dura mater are manifested as constriction at joints. Erratic movement between two bones eventually causes a pattern of constriction and irregular movement throughout the cranium.

Fundamental Concepts: Dysfunction and Direction of Ease

The conventional manner of studying irregular motion among the bones of the cranial base is in terms of "dysfunction." Each movement is classified by its apparent deviation from an ideal or standard. A release procedure is tailored to each dysfunction. This approach is based on a medical model of healing. Symptoms specify a diagnosis. Each diagnosis requires a unique intervention.

In practice, the movement of the sphenoid is not so simply expressed by these classical categories. The sphenoid contacts every other bone in the cranial vault. Each pattern of movement that we encounter is the result of a complex set of forces that act on the sphenoid and its sutures. Thus, sphenoid motion reflects movement and restriction of all the surrounding bones.

Despite the oversimplification, the conventional model is useful for learning. This system of classification alerts the practitioner to a variety of possibilities. Knowing and practicing the examples presented in the following material, the therapist gains familiarity with movements and relationships within the cranial base. She develops confidence in her understanding of the information communicated through the hands.

This classification is based on the work of Dr. William Sutherland. Because of the key position of the sphenoid, he categorized irregularities in terms of sphenoid movement. Further, he considered that the problem rested in that unique joint between occiput and sphenoid, the sphenobasilar synchondrosis. Subsequent experience has shown that this is not the complete picture.

The sphenobasilar synchondrosis probably does not hold these restrictions, but rather adapts to them. In other words, the combination of restriction and of flexibility in the interaction of all the bones around the sphenoid influences its alignment. This alignment impacts its joint with the occiput and puts a special stamp on its movement. Thus, it mimics a specific dysfunction. Nevertheless, I follow Sutherland's system of naming here, as his recognition of nuances of movement is useful, even if it is based on a different understanding of the origin of those movements.

Furthermore, Sutherland's model offers an important conceptualization of the release process: movement in the direction of ease. Its chief tenet is not to fight against or force an apparent restriction, but to work with it. This leads to a greater understanding of and appreciation for the body's adaptive mechanism. We learn again to work with the body's capabilities, following its path, rather than to impose our own.

This chapter presents the dysfunctions in order of severity of symptoms, specifying the symptoms and the release procedure for each dysfunction. The final dysfunction and release, compression-decompression, will be familiar from the basic course. Though it can be very severe, a mild compression is also common among clients. It is usually associated with tight back muscles and a generalized restriction in the craniosacral rhythm. The compression-decompression release of the sphenoid is usually effective in the release of the other dysfunctions.

The Importance of the Cranial Base

Around the cranial base are many openings (foramina) through the dura mater and the bone. The largest is the foramen magnum. By allowing the passage of arteries, veins, and nerves, the foramina form a link in the paths of communication between the cranial vault and all that is beyond it. Any unusual restriction of the dura mater or misalignment of bones may disturb normal flow of fluid or nerve impulse through these important openings. The results can be fluid pressure buildup, lack of proper drainage, and interference with nerve and endocrine function.

The cranial base is not merely the floor of a protective case; it is rather a dynamic, interactive structure, intimately linked with the bones, muscle,

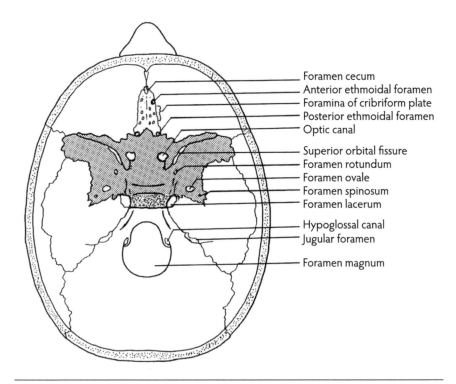

Foramen cecum
Anterior ethmoidal foramen
Foramina of cribriform plate
Posterior ethmoidal foramen
Optic canal

Superior orbital fissure
Foramen rotundum
Foramen ovale
Foramen spinosum
Foramen lacerum

Hypoglossal canal
Jugular foramen

Foramen magnum

Figure 61. Some of the Foramina of the Cranial Base. These passageways provide for communication and flow between the cranial vault and the entire body.

and nerve and connective tissue of the face, neck, and shoulders. By way of the blood vessels and nerves that pass through the cranial base, the brain and the entire body are in communication.

The Rhythmic Motion: Flexion and Extension

Because the first neck vertebra supports the occiput, and the base of the occiput in turn supports the base of the sphenoid, both these cranial bones move together with a rocking motion. However, the therapist feels the motion more simply. On the sphenoid, occiput, and other bones of the cranial vault, the chief components of movement are *outward* and *inward*. Components of this motion are felt throughout the skull, and along the spine to the sacrum. The shoulders and legs also appear to move in resonance with the cranial impulse.

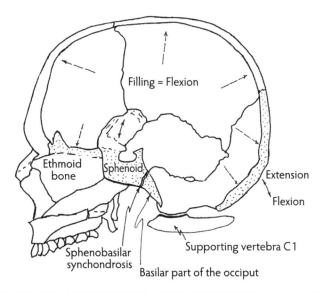

Figure 62. Motions of Flexion and Extension. Flexing around the relatively stable platform provided by the cervical spine, cranial bones press outward in every direction with increasing pressure due to production of cerebrospinal fluid. The direction of the occipital bone is back and down. The direction of the sphenoid is mainly downward. These bones must bend away from the center of the cranial vault at their common joint, the sphenobasilar synchondrosis. During extension, with absorption of cerebrospinal fluid the motion is reversed. Double-headed arrows on sphenoid and at occiput indicate this cyclical motion.

Therapists have attempted to explain the motion of the bones of the cranium and the spine in this way: As cerebrospinal fluid is produced, pressure in the skull increases, pushing the enveloping structure outward in every direction. The cranial sutures expand slightly. At some point, a signal reaches the ventricles, and production of fluid is curtailed.

As cerebrospinal fluid is absorbed in the arachnoid villi and throughout the system, pressure within the cranium decreases. The vault contracts, as each of the sutures closes slightly.

A century ago, William Sutherland named these motions for the apparent action at the sphenobasilar synchondrosis. Because the expansive, outward thrust is associated with a bending at the sphenobasilar joint, this phase of the rhythm is known as *flexion.*

As pressure in the cranium decreases during absorption and the entire vault contracts, the sphenoid and occipital bones tilt upward and inward on this same hinge. Sutherland called this motion *extension.*

We often apply these terms to any motion related to the craniosacral rhythm. Flexion refers to any motion throughout the body that is associated with the "filling" part of the cycle. Extension refers to any motion related to the "emptying" part, while fluid is being absorbed and pressure decreasing. This use causes confusion at first because most other body parts appear to be spreading (extending) as the joint between sphenoid and occiput is flexing. Nevertheless, the phases of the cranial rhythm anywhere in the body are named for the motion between sphenoid and occiput.

To rephrase, during flexion, or filling, the sphenoid presses downward. We palpate this movement at the temples, which cover the greater wings of the sphenoid. The occiput moves outward and downward, levering over the cervical spine. These bones are joined by a cartilage hinge, the sphenobasilar synchondrosis.

During extension, or absorption, the sphenoid moves upward; the occiput moves inward and upward.

Release in the Direction of Ease: The Indirect Method

Put simply, physiological movement often appears to be easy in one direction and restricted in the other. To push against the restriction is to work *directly.* For example, stretching a tight muscle pushes directly against the contraction. When a restriction is chronic or painful, this often stimulates resistance in the affected tissue, and it may cause greater discomfort.

Moving in the direction that is easier and more comfortable is working *indirectly.* We gently follow the inclination embedded in the tissue. This appears to offer support and relief to physiological structures that have been caught up in an unrewarding effort. The area can then relax its effort and seek a new balance. Many forms of therapy have discovered that moving in the direction of ease aids the release of restrictions, restoring balance and symmetry.

Compensatory Dysfunctions of the Cranial Base

These first four dysfunctions—flexion, extension, torsion, and side bending—are usually associated with, even caused by, constriction and misalignment in the body. The body compensates by developing a way to move around a restriction. Muscle and fascia reorganize to produce a new alignment that eventually extends throughout the body. This compensatory alignment follows muscle and fascia through the neck, communicating an imbalance at the cranial base.

When we discover one of these cranial base dysfunctions, it underscores the importance of releasing restrictions throughout the body.

Flexion Dysfunction

The sphenoid, as palpated at the greater wings, appears to move further or more strongly downward during the filling or expansion phase of the craniosacral rhythm.

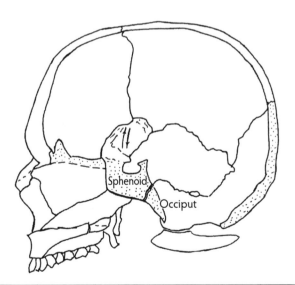

Figure 63. Flexion or Extension Dysfunction. The greater wings of the sphenoid move more fully into flexion (downward) or extension (upward) during each cycle of the craniosacral rhythm.

Extension Dysfunction

The sphenoid, as palpated at the greater wings, appears to move further or more strongly upward during the absorption or contraction phase of the craniosacral rhythm.

Symptoms

Both flexion and extension dysfunctions are sometimes associated with recurrent headaches, sinus problems, and low back pain. The severity of symptoms may vary from mild to moderate.

Self-palpation

You may palpate the craniosacral rhythm on yourself by bringing your hands to the sides of your head. Place the end pad of each little finger over your temple, contacting the greater wings of the sphenoid. Bring the end pad of each thumb around behind your head to rest on the occiput, where neck muscles attach. If this position is too awkward for comfort, you may approximate it by touching each thumb to the mastoid process, just behind the ears. Let yourself become quiet. Rather than focusing on your hands, bring your attention inward to your center. As you let yourself drop expectations and effort, you will become attuned to the subtle motion of the bones. Notice whether the greater wings move downward along with the downward and outward motion of the occiput (and a downward rotation of the mastoid process). The greater wings move upward while the occiput moves upward and inward (and the mastoid process rotates upward).

Often the motions we palpate vary from the theoretical ideal. This is natural. Minor constrictions of connective tissue in the torso, shoulders, neck, or head give a unique coloring to the rhythmic motion characteristic of each of us. In this self-palpation, note whether the movement in one direction appears fuller, longer, or easier than the other. If so, this is the direction of "dysfunction."

Client Palpation and Assessment

To palpate this rhythm on your client, ask him or her to lie face upward on a padded treatment table. Sit at the head of the table, resting your forearms and elbows on the table. It is helpful to use a chair that is low enough so that you are not hanging over the client's face as you work. Bring your hands to each side of the client's head so that your thumbs comfortably contact the temples, just behind the corner of each eye. Slide the little finger of each hand slightly under the base of the skull. If your little fingers cannot extend under the back of the head let them rest as far as they reach. Beneath the pads of your thumbs, covered by muscle, are the broad extensions known as the greater wings of the sphenoid.

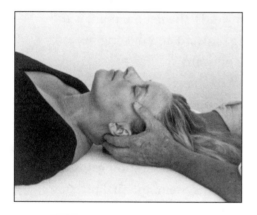

Figure 64a. Hand Position at the Sphenoid.

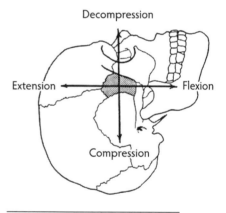

Figure 64b. Sphenoid Movement.

The hand position for assessing and releasing the dysfunctions of the cranial base is the same as that used for the sphenoid decompression. The hands are brought to the sides of the head so that the pads of the thumbs can comfortably contact the greater wings of the sphenoid. The soft tissue commonly known as the temple covers the wings. The position is just behind the corner of the eye and above the zygomatic arch. The palms and fingers lightly cradle the head, with little fingers at the occiput, if they will comfortably reach. The diagram shows the motions of flexion and extension contrasted with the directions for the compression-decompression release.

Attend to the movement of the sphenoid and the occiput. Generally you will feel them moving downward (flexion) or upward (extension) together. Imagine they are hinging at their joint and bending around the stabilizing fulcrum of the atlas, the first cervical vertebra.

Notice variations in the cycle of the craniosacral rhythm, especially in the sphenoid. Does one direction appear stronger or longer than the other? How smooth is the movement? If there is a difference, is it in the direction of flexion or of extension?

The Neutral Zone

Sometimes, therapists conceptualize a "neutral zone" in the craniosacral rhythm. Imagine that the rhythm is divided into segments. Each segment is one cycle. A cycle includes one flexion and one extension. The neutral point is the point of presumed equilibrium between the motion of flexion and the motion of extension. In other words, the neutral point is the instant between our perception of moving outward and moving inward, and between moving inward and moving outward.

The term *neutral* is based on the theory of changing pressures within the vault. As fluid pressure increases, cranial bones are pressed outward from the center. The dura mater stretches as space at the sutures expands, until a point at which a signal is given to halt production. With the stopping of fluid production, the continuing process of absorption gains the upper hand. Fluid is absorbed into the vascular system, internal pressure begins to drop, and the cranial bones begin to move inward. As the cranial vault contracts, the dura mater and the tissue at the sutures again pass through a zone of greater ease and harmony. As internal fluid pressure continues to decrease, the cranial bones move closer at their sutures, until they reach the point of greatest contact and pressure at the sutures. Again, a physiological signal is given, fluid production resumes, and internal fluid pressure causes a renewed expansion of the cranial vault.

This concept of a neutral zone, a condition of relative ease at the endpoint of each process of expansion or contraction, may be helpful in describing the relative quality of movement on each side of the rhythmic cycle. For instance, it may assist in deciding whether the client's craniosacral rhythm manifests a flexion or extension dysfunction.

Releasing Procedure

We treat flexion or extension dysfunctions by following the sphenoid in its full range of motion, accentuating slightly the dysfunctional direction. Continue until you experience signs of a therapeutic release, especially a feeling of ease and broadening in the craniosacral rhythm.

Torsion Dysfunction

Torsion is a tilting of the sphenoid. Looking directly at the client's face, the sphenoid with its greater wings tends to tilt either clockwise or counterclockwise. Of course, the degree of tilt or torsion is very small. But it is accompanied by disturbances of pressure and motion along the sutures of the sphenoid with the other cranial bones.

Symptoms

The degree of torsion varies, as does the severity of symptoms. The client may suffer from allergies, headaches, and neck or back pain. Eye coordination problems have been observed. The sacrum may tilt in the same direction as the sphenoid.

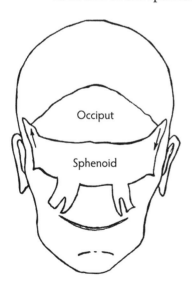

Figure 65. Torsion. This is a tendency of the sphenoid to tilt clockwise or counterclockwise in relation to other cranial bones, as palpated at the greater wings of the sphenoid. The torsion is named for the side on which the greater wing is superior. Here, a right torsion dysfunction is shown.

Self-palpation

You can gain a greater understanding of torsion by palpating it on yourself. Bringing your hands to the sides of your face, place your third or fourth fingers over the greater wings of the sphenoid at each temple. Lightly holding your face with the palms of your hands, monitor the craniosacral rhythm at the temples. Now exert a light clockwise or counterclockwise pressure by drawing one of the greater wings upward and the other downward. Note the degree of response in your sphenoid to this unusual motion. Next, exert a light pressure in the opposite direction on each side of the sphenoid at the temples, downward and upward. Allow time for the bones to respond to each movement. Afterward, monitor your rhythm as the motion of your sphenoid returns to normal.

Client Assessment

From a sitting position, place your hands as described previously, with thumb pads at the temples and little fingers near the occiput. Stabilize the occiput by a constant, light contact with the little fingers. Then gently press the greater wing downward (toward the feet) with one thumb, while drawing upward (toward the top of the head) with the other thumb.

Test in each direction. Allow time for the bones to respond to each movement. If the movement is the same, tilting to the same degree in each direction, then torsion is not a problem for this client. If the movement is greater in one direction, then there is a torsion dysfunction.

The dysfunction is named for the side on which the greater wing tends to move higher. For example, a right torsion dysfunction is one in which the sphenoid allows greater range of motion tilting with the client's right side high and the left side low.

Releasing Procedure

With your hands in the same positions as above, gently move the sphenoid in the direction of ease (into the dysfunction) until a release occurs. Test for greater excursion in the opposite direction after the release and for greater freedom in the normal cycle of the craniosacral rhythm.

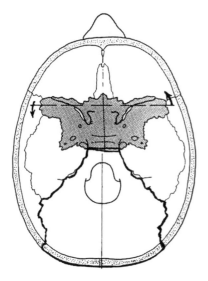

Figure 66. Side Bending. The greater wings of the sphenoid twist back toward the occiput on one side of the head, away from the occiput on the other side. The dysfunction is named for the convexity associated with the anterior movement of the greater wing. Shown here: side bending with right convexity.

Side Bending Dysfunction

Side bending is a condition in which the sphenoid and the occiput tend to twist right or left toward each other, hinging sideways on the cartilage pad at their joint.

Symptoms

The symptoms observed are similar to those found with torsion.

Self-palpation

You can get a sense of this motion on yourself. Place your hands at the sides of your head, with little fingers over the greater wings at the temples and thumbs hooked around to the occiput behind your head. Notice the craniosacral rhythm as both thumbs and little fingers move upward or downward together.

Now apply a slight posterior pressure with the little finger on one side, drawing the little finger toward the thumb at the occiput. Do you feel a response in the greater wing of the sphenoid? Repeat with the hand on the other side. Then allow the rhythm to return to normal. This movement of greater wing toward occiput on the same side is side bending. It is named for the side on which the greater wing moves anteriorly.

Client Assessment

Sitting with your client as before, monitor the craniosacral rhythm in sphenoid and occiput with the thumb and little finger of each hand. While stabilizing the occiput with your little fingers, apply a slight side bending pressure, drawing the greater wing of the sphenoid toward the occiput on one side. Note the apparent ease and degree of movement. Release the pressure, wait a few moments for the cranial system to balance itself, and apply a similar pressure with the hand on the other side. Note the apparent ease and degree of movement on this side.

If the apparent degree of movement is greater on one side than the other, there is a side bending dysfunction in the cranial base of your client.

While holding the sphenoid and occiput in a side bend, you may sense a concavity or emptiness on the side you are pressing, with a convexity or fullness on the other side. Technically, for professional communication or treatment notes, this dysfunction is called *side bending, with right (or left) convexity.*

However, the *direction of ease* is the side of concavity, the side on which the greater wing approaches the occiput more closely.

Releasing Procedure

This dysfunction is released by moving the sphenoid gently into the side bending dysfunction that you discovered in your assessment and holding it lightly until you notice signs of release, especially a sense of widening, relaxing, easing. Then test both directions of side bending again to confirm that the dysfunction is released and distance in each direction is equal.

Intracranial Dysfunctions: Strain and Compression

The previous dysfunctions were adjustments to muscular and postural imbalance reaching upward from the body. We usually consider that the following three dysfunctions—lateral strain, vertical strain, and compression—are the result of a head injury. In that case, the symptoms may be serious. However, sometimes there is no memory of an injury, yet restrictions within the cranium mimic these dysfunctions. The symptoms are not as severe. As we will see, compression between the sphenoid and the basilar portion of the occiput is often associated with other compressions along the spinal column.

Lateral Strain Dysfunction

In side bending, one side tends to twist back, the other forward, hinging at the sphenobasilar synchondrosis. In lateral strain, the entire sphenoid appears to have shifted to one side. This places a strain on the sphenobasilar synchondrosis. A blow to the side of the head may have caused this lateral shift.

Symptoms

Severe lateral strain has been observed in association with chronic headaches and personality disturbance. Learning disabilities and strabismus in children and spastic cerebral palsy may occur. The sphenoid may bulge at the temple.

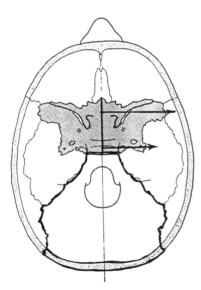

Figure 67. Lateral Strain. The entire sphenoid appears to shift sideways, straining the cartilage at the sphenobasilar joint. Here, arrows indicate the direction of displacement in a right lateral strain.

Do not assume that these severe symptoms will always occur. We often notice apparent lateral strain with none of these symptoms.

Self-palpation

To gain familiarity with this motion on yourself, place your hands at the sides of your face, with third or fourth fingers over the greater wings of the sphenoid. Allow yourself time to sense that you are in contact with the sphenoid bone. Then press inward on one side, in the direction of the opposite wing. On the other side, draw the greater wing forward (anteriorly). This causes the body of the sphenoid to displace sideways and introduces sideways strain at the sphenobasilar synchondrosis.

Note the degree or the feel of this displacement. Then return to center and move the sphenoid sideways in the other direction. Note the degree of displacement. Use very light pressure and return to center if the motion becomes uncomfortable. When finished, monitor your craniosacral rhythm as it resumes. If the sphenoid moved more easily or further to one side, it may indicate a lateral strain in that direction.

Client Assessment

To assess lateral strain on your client, maintain the position used for the previous dysfunctions, with your thumbs on the greater wings of the sphenoid and your little fingers stabilizing the occiput. After establishing contact and monitoring the rhythm, move the sphenoid laterally. Press very lightly inward (medially) on the greater wing with one thumb, while supporting the opposite wing and drawing it anteriorly. This contact and support with the other thumb is necessary to move the body of the sphenoid to the side and prevent it twisting back as in side bending.

Note the degree of displacement. Then repeat the process, displacing the sphenoid laterally from the opposite side.

A lateral strain dysfunction is present if the sphenoid displaces more to one side than to the other. The dysfunction is named for the direction of ease of displacement.

Releasing Procedure

Displace the sphenoid laterally in the direction of ease, in the same manner in which you assessed the dysfunction. For example, if the sphenoid moved easier, or further, when pressed from left to right, then you have discovered a right lateral strain. Release by again displacing the sphenoid from left to right and holding until you feel a sense of widening and easing. Test in the other direction. Then remain present and monitor the sphenoid as the craniosacral rhythm returns.

Vertical Strain Dysfunction

In vertical strain, the body of the sphenoid is displaced either higher (superior vertical strain) or lower (inferior vertical strain) at the sphenobasilar synchondrosis.

Superior vertical strain is associated with a tilting forward and downward at the greater wings of the sphenoid. With inferior vertical strain the greater wings of the sphenoid tend to tilt upward.

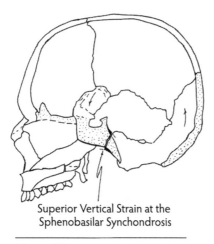
Superior Vertical Strain at the
Sphenobasilar Synchondrosis

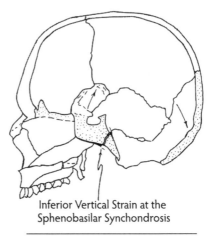
Inferior Vertical Strain at the
Sphenobasilar Synchondrosis

Figure 68a.
Superior Vertical Strain.

Figure 68b.
Inferior Vertical Strain.

The body of the sphenoid is slightly superior or inferior at its joint with the basilar portion of the occiput. Arrows on the sphenoid and occiput indicate the direction of release for each condition.

Symptoms

Vertical strain originates with trauma to the head affecting the intracranial membranes and the sutures. The trauma may occur during birth, or it may occur later in life. It may be a blow to the front or the back of the head. Severe vertical strain occurs independently of restrictions in the body. However, chronic displacements in the cranium may eventually reflect downward to the musculature and posture of the body.

Vertical strain is a serious condition that may lead to chronic, severe headache. Unusual patterns of head and facial pain may be present.

Due to displacements within the cranial vault, the slope of the forehead may be affected. A superior vertical strain may cause the forehead to bulge forward at the top. An inferior vertical strain may cause the forehead to slope back from the brows to the top.

Palpation of vertical strain on yourself is not recommended.

Assessment

The position of therapist and client is as described for all the previous cranial base dysfunctions. The therapist stabilizes the occiput and assesses movement of the sphenoid, as for flexion/extension dysfunction. However, in testing for vertical strain the therapist adds some pressure at each extreme, drawing the greater wings more fully into flexion and into extension.

If the sphenoid goes more fully downward into flexion, in the presence of other symptoms, then a superior vertical strain at the sphenobasilar junction is assumed.

If the sphenoid goes more fully upward into extension, in the presence of other symptoms, then an inferior vertical strain is assumed.

Releasing Procedure

This procedure is similar to that described for flexion and extension dysfunctions. Move the sphenoid in the direction of ease and gently hold until there is a sense of release and widening. Follow any small movement until a full release is felt.

If there is no release, then the occiput may also be utilized. For superior vertical strain, as you move the greater wings downward into flexion, draw the occiput upward into extension. For inferior vertical strain, as you move the greater wings upward into extension, draw the occiput downward into flexion. As usual, use light pressure, a gentle touch, and plenty of patience in attempting to release this painful dysfunction.

Compression Dysfunction

Compression dysfunction is a condition in which intracranial restrictions result in the compression of the sphenoid back against the basilar portion of the occiput, compressing their common juncture. There is a tendency for this to occur in mild form in many people. It is often associated with compression at the atlanto-occipital joint and at the point where the spine joins the sacrum, L5/S1. There is a lack of flexibility and responsiveness throughout the dura mater, giving a sense of compression throughout the spine and cranium.

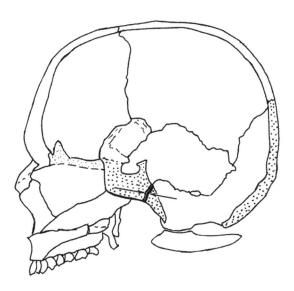

Figure 69. Compression at the Sphenobasilar Synchondrosis.

Symptoms

These forms of compression limit overall flexibility. When they are present in mild form, the client seems to feel constricted and dissatisfied regarding life choices. The client will often put a lot of energy into pondering the problems in his or her life, with no apparent resolution or change. In a more serious form, these compressions have been found to be associated with severe depression.

Assessment and Release

We assess compression through observation during the release procedure. This is the compression-decompression release of the sphenoid taught in the basic course of craniosacral therapy.

The preceding exercises have sensitized you, as therapist, to the various dysfunctions possible in the cranial base. With that background, the compression-decompression release will assume new dimensions. As the sphenoid, by means of its greater wings, is compressed against the base of the occiput, it may be felt to move in the manner of torsion, side bending, or strain. Both compression and decompression may serve to reveal these dysfunctional tendencies. In each instance the therapist follows into the direction of ease, while maintaining the compressing or decompressing pressure. Consequently, the compression-decompression release of the sphenoid serves to also release most components of the other cranial base dysfunctions.

To perform the compression release, maintain your previous position. The client is lying face up on the padded table. You are sitting at the head, your forearms resting on the table, hands at the sides of the client's head. The thumb pad of each hand is contacting the greater wing of the sphenoid at the temple. Your little fingers contact the occiput.

Beneath the skin and muscle tissue on each side, you are contacting the bony structure of the sphenoid's greater wing. As you become centered and still, you will perceive components of the craniosacral rhythm. Silently recommend a movement back, toward the occiput and the fingerlike projections of the temporal bone, into the cranial base. Traditionally, this is considered compression into the sphenobasilar synchondrosis. Pressure is not necessary. Rather, maintain a persistent presence and alertness. Giving space and freedom, follow the movement in a posterior direction. Often, you will notice many variations from a symmetrical movement, such as torsion and side bending.

More than one indication of release may be felt as the sphenoid moves, then halts and moves again. All the sutures along the sphenoid are being exercised, and many areas of constriction may be addressed during both phases of this release. When the sphenoid seems to rest quietly, to have found a "floor" to its posterior movement, you are ready to begin the second phase. Often there is a feeling of widening at the occiput.

Maintaining the same finger positions and internal space, gently recommend a motion forward, toward the connections of the sphenoid with the frontal bone and the face. Traditionally this is known as the decompression phase, with respect to the sphenobasilar synchondrosis. As the sphenoid moves forward, accept all the variations from symmetrical motion. Maintain your contact and intent through brief periods of no apparent movement. Be sensitive to sensations of energy release or a side-to-side fluctuation of energy that tells you the dura mater is actively unwinding even when you feel no sign of movement in the sphenoid.

The release is complete when there is a sense of relaxation and broadening, and the craniosacral rhythm returns evenly and fully.

Completion and Follow-up

Practice of these assessment and release procedures sensitizes you to the variety of dysfunctional movements imposed on the sphenoid by constrictions throughout the cranial vault. As you gain sensitivity, you will be able to assess and assist in the release of most restrictions through the sphenoid compression-decompression.

When you encounter a client with severe, chronic head pain, you will be alerted to assess carefully for strain or compression and to follow up over several sessions.

It may take more than one session to obtain full release of a severe dysfunction that has been going on for a long time. The entire system needs time to adapt, even to constructive change. Thus it is more beneficial to assist in the beginning of change than to become frustrated attempting to force a complete correction in a single session.

The Temporal Bones

Freedom of movement and synchronization of rhythm in the temporal bones are an important component of cranial functioning. The ear pull technique helps release restrictions in the sutures and the dura mater. The mastoid and three-finger techniques are helpful in restoring synchronization and a full range to the craniosacral rhythm.

When these techniques seem inadequate, then look more carefully at the occiput and the quality of muscle and connective tissue reaching upward through the neck. A holding within the connective tissue around the cranial base is often in response to a chronic pulling by muscle and ligament reaching upward from the shoulders and chest.

The Occiput

The method of inducing a still point at the occiput (Sutherland called it the CV4 technique) also serves to release the occiput at its sutures with the parietal and temporal bones. This can be helpful early in the treatment when the entire cranial base is very constricted.

The Pelvis

After completing these releases of the membranes and sutures of the cranial vault, it is instructive and helpful to return to the pelvic area. Assess the sacrum for balance and freedom of movement at the end of that session, or in a separate session within a few days.

Chapter 9

Releasing the Bones of the Mouth and the Face

In beginning the study of craniosacral therapy, we moved from the body and the spinal column to the cranial vault, focusing on this enclosed system of bone, membrane, fluid, and nerve tissue. Now we expand our attention outward from the cranial vault to appraise the functioning of the entire cranium, including the mouth and the face.

The skull as a mere protective case could be a hard and rigid container, like a seashell. Instead, it is a flexible structure, composed of interwoven segments and layers. The facial bones are built outward and downward from the vault in a variety of shapes adapted to unique life functions. The strength and flexibility of the cranial vault extends to the face and to the apparatus of mastication (chewing).

The bones that make up the cranial vault and the face are not isolated from one another, but intimately related. There is a harmony of function and interconnection, of integration, that exceeds almost anything humans have devised or envisioned. Within the body it is the flexibility and interconnection of structures and functions that make for effectiveness, responsiveness, and the ability to recover from injury.

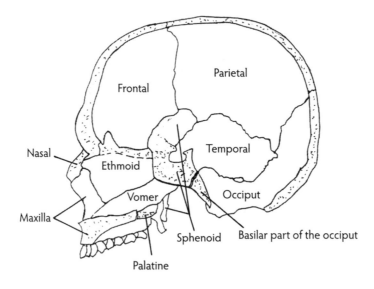

Figure 70. The Bones of the Cranial Vault, the Face, and the Mouth.

The head as a whole supports complex functions, such as nonverbal and nonconscious perception, assessment, and response; conscious perception, thought, and communication; as well as basic life functions such as sucking, chewing, swallowing, spitting, and breathing. The activities of the head have meaning only in connection with the information, fluids, and multifaceted functioning of the entire body. Though the cranial vault fascinates us because of its special structure and because it protects the brain, it is misleading to rank body parts or functions as higher, lower, noble, or base. Sucking takes place in close proximity to the organ of abstract thinking. A running nose has an impact on the keenest vision. The awareness conveyed through the senses of smell, taste, and touch brings a quality to our life that is on a par with and colors the most profound thought or artistic vision.

The Mouth, Face, and Jaw

In this chapter, we will consider the following components of the cranium:

- the maxillas, the two bones that form most of the upper jaw and also provide a framework for the face;

- the vomer, a thin plate separating the nasal passages, which establishes an inner bridge between the sphenoid and the roof of the mouth;

- the palatines, two delicate bones sandwiched between the sphenoid and the maxillas that also form part of the hard palate;

- the zygomas, the cheekbones below the outer corner of each eye;

- the teeth;

- the nasal bones, forming the bridge of the nose; and

- the ethmoid bone, a part of the cranial vault between the eyes and below the frontal bone.

Craniosacral therapists often call this region of the cranium the *hard palate* because of the attention given to the maxillas and the palatines. Together these bones form the roof of the mouth, the hard palate.

Most of these bones directly join the bones of the cranial vault. But none forms a part of the vault or is embedded in the dura mater. The rhythmical movement of these mouth and face bones is propelled by their contact with the cranial bones. Conversely, conditions of freedom or restriction within this structure influence the flexibility of the cranial vault.

The mouth and the face are areas of special sensitivity. It is largely through the senses of the mouth that the newborn begins to explore and know the world. Senses of smell, vision, and hearing join taste and touch to contribute important aspects of our "feel" of the world in which we live. Lingering pain and dysfunction in the face or mouth can seriously dampen our life appreciation and our sense of proportion in making sense of our world. An injury to the face may result in a contraction of connective tissue and restriction of movement among the bones. Nerve and fluid pathways become constricted, causing pain and lack of symmetry that may continue long after apparent healing.

Life stress also has an influence on the comfort and functioning of this region. The mouth and face comprise an important avenue of interaction with our world. We express much of the self through both words and appearance. This region may be affected by the unconscious activities of clenching and grinding of the teeth. More subtly, significant regions may be affected by constriction of muscles and connective tissue. This constriction may have a profound effect on personal comfort as well as muscle and nerve functioning.

The bones and muscles of the mouth and face have an important impact on the bones of the cranial vault. The maxilla bones, which form the face and upper jaw, directly join the frontal and ethmoid bones of the cranial vault and indirectly interface with the sphenoid through the vomer and the palatine bones. Any misalignment of the maxillas due to injury may influence the alignment and the rhythmical motion of these cranial bones.

In addition, the maxillas articulate with every other facial bone except the lower jaw. And they are in intimate and constant contact with that bone through the teeth.

The lower jaw, the mandible, is a common focus of pain and restricted motion. Muscles of chewing originate on the frontal, sphenoid, and temporal bones. Any misalignment of the mandible repeatedly transmits an unbalancing force to these bones. Habitual clenching and grinding of the teeth speaks of constricting, compressing, and levering forces exerted on the mandible, the maxillas, the sphenoid, and the temporal bones.

The entire structure of the cranial vault, the jaw, and the face is intimately connected through sutures, fascia, and the cyclical motion of the craniosacral rhythm. So it is seldom that any source of pain or restriction is limited to the area in which it is felt. For most effective relief, the entire interactive structure needs to be considered. For practical purposes we first release or balance the foundation of the face: the sphenoid, frontal, and temporal bones. Then we investigate the larger bones that form the framework: the mandible and the maxillas. The vomer is added because of its importance as a connector and transmitter of movement. The smaller palatine, nasal, and zygomatic bones will often balance themselves if the maxillas, the vomer, the sphenoid, and the temporal bones have been relieved of restrictions.

The Bones and Their Natural Rhythmic Motions

The sphenoid, frontal, ethmoid, and temporal bones all contact facial bones and transmit some component of the craniosacral rhythm. The sphenoid transmits a down and upward motion to the bones and tissue it contacts. Because the frontal joins the sphenoid all across the cranial base, the frontal also shares in this downward and upward motion that

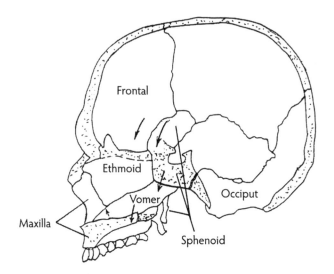

Figure 71. Response of Vomer and Maxillas to the Craniosacral Rhythm.
Arrows show forces exerted on the frontal, sphenoid, and vomer bones
with the production of cerebrospinal fluid, during flexion. The motions
of absorption or extension are in the opposite directions.

is clearly palpable on either bone. Yet, the frontal can also be felt to swell forward as it moves downward with the "filling" of the cranial vault.

Nestled just behind the nasal bones, the ethmoid makes a small but important contribution to the floor of the cranial vault. Each side of its upper surface is attached to the frontal, and it reaches back to join the sphenoid. Situated as it is, the ethmoid also shares in the downward-upward motion of frontal and sphenoid.

During the flexion or filling phase of the cycle, the sphenoid presses downward on the upper, posterior portion of the vomer. Probably the perpendicular plate of the ethmoid joins in exerting a slight downward pressure on the long upper edge of the vomer.

The vomer, flaring at its base to join the maxillas and cap their mid-sagittal suture, transmits a downward thrust to the hard palate between the molars. The arched roof of the mouth flattens slightly with each flexion, spreading the gums and molars to the side. On extension the sphenoid and the vomer rise, drawing upward on the roof of the mouth, drawing the gums and molars toward the middle. These motions can be palpated on the teeth or gums and on the midline of the hard palate.

The two palatine bones are roughly L-shaped. They help to form the inner roof of the mouth and the inner nasal passages. The horizontal plates of the palatine bones continue the arched roof of the mouth behind the maxillas. Like the maxillas, they join at the center of the hard palate. The downward-upward thrust of the vomer can also be felt on the central ridge between the palatines.

The perpendicular plate extends upward from each palatine on the outer sides of the nasal passage. It is sandwiched between the sphenoid and the maxilla, forming a vertical buffer or gasket between them. This perpendicular segment of the palatine bone reaches all the way up to the orbit of the eye to form a part of its floor. The down-and-up motion of the sphenoid is more of a friction than a pressing on the shared vertical joints and membranes across the palatines to the maxillas. Because of the delicacy of these bones, we do not attempt to coordinate with the craniosacral rhythm when we release the palatines, but only to enhance freedom of movement.

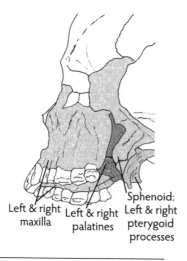

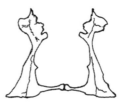

Left & right palatines
from behind

Figure 72a. The Position of the Palatines.

Figure 72b. The Palatines from Behind.

The palatine bones form a gasket between the sphenoid and the maxilla. Each bone extends from its horizontal plate in the hard palate upward to a point deep in the orbit of the eye where it contributes to the floor of the eye socket. The form of the palatine is actually finer and more complex than depicted here.

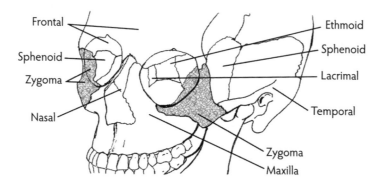

Figure 73. The Bones of the Face. The long, thin nasal bones cap the nasal passage. The zygomatic arch extends from the zygoma to the temporal bone, forming a bridge over the muscles reaching from the lower jaw.

The nasal bones are thin plates that lie against the upper part of the maxillas to form the bridge of the nose. The upper end of each bone joins the frontal bone, and inwardly they touch the perpendicular plate of the ethmoid. Their rhythmic movement reflects the complex outward and downward motion of the frontal, ethmoid, and maxilla bones. Again, in releasing we enhance freedom of movement rather than attempt to coordinate with the craniosacral rhythm.

The zygomatic bones, or cheekbones, are at the corner of each eye. They join the frontal above and the maxilla beneath to contribute to the orbit of the eye. They also join the greater wing of the sphenoid at the temple. The zygoma bridges across the musculature of chewing to join the temporal bone and form the zygomatic arch. These bones give the characteristic shape to a person's cheeks. If they are compressed into their sutures, they may drag on the motion of the other bones involved. The release of even a minor restriction in the zygomatic bones often feels wonderful to the client because of the great sensitivity of the face to any stress.

Self-palpation

This is most effective if you are able to look at the bone structure in an anatomical atlas or use the drawings in this book as you explore your own face. In addition, notice the feelings stirred up in you as you touch your mouth and face.

Vomer

Begin with a finger inside the mouth. The ridge along the midline at the roof of the mouth corresponds to the suture between the left and right maxilla and the left and right palatine bones. Hold your finger lightly against this ridge between the molars. You may sense the craniosacral rhythm, transmitted by the vomer. The motion is downward on flexion and upward on extension.

Palatine Bones

The maxilla bone on each side of the midline suture provides a foundation for the gums and the bed out of which grow the teeth. Find your last molar on one side and slide your finger inward or medially to the roof. If the last molar (the wisdom tooth) has been removed, you will find a platform on the gums behind the last tooth. Move medially from this platform. This is the location of the palatine bones. They nestle behind the maxillas, extending the hard palate between the gum platforms, which reach around them on each side.

Maxillas

Place the backs of two fingers lightly against the upper molars and relax your lower jaw. Support that arm with the other so that you can rest quietly and comfortably for a few moments. You may be able to feel the widening and narrowing of the hard palate as the pressure of the vomer changes the shape of the roof of the mouth.

Zygomas

Now bring one finger to the outside of the upper teeth, still inside the cheek. Following your gum line back, you will notice a bony structure directly above your finger as you reach the molars. The maxilla flares out on each side, then gives way to the zygomatic bone, which it supports. Find the zygomatic bone from outside with your other hand. Feel the contour of the zygoma between the fingers. Further back along the gums and the cheek, you can feel a muscle from the lower jaw reaching upward to pass beneath the zygomatic arch. Palpate the motion of the muscle from inside, moving your jaw open and closed.

Teeth

Now lightly grasp your teeth between thumb and forefinger. Slowly palpate around the teeth from back to front on each side. Notice the changing sensations associated with this gentle touch.

Maxillas from Outside

Continue your explorations outside the mouth. With the fingers of both hands on the upper lips, follow the structure of upper teeth and gums back on each side until you feel the cheekbones flare outward. The foundation of this structure is the maxilla on each side. The prominence, however large or small, angular or straight, is formed by the zygoma.

Now return your fingers to your upper lips. Follow the underlying structure of the maxilla on each side upward, beside the nose, to the orbit of the eye. The maxilla forms the bony frame of the eye socket just inward of the bridge of the nose and for almost half of the distance under the eye. Carefully follow this ridge from the inner corner of the eye and along the base of the socket.

Zygomas from Outside

The outer base and side of the eye socket is formed by the zygoma. Continue following the orbit of the eye. Then palpate the zygoma as it forms a ridge just below the outer corner of the eye and carries the line around the side of the face. Joining the temporal bone, it contributes to the zygomatic arch. Palpate this, following back to the ear canal.

Bring one finger of each hand to the lower orbit of each eye. Gently feel along this edge, below the eye, attempting to sense the location of the suture where maxilla and zygoma join. Follow the suture line downward and outward diagonally, then curve to the back on each side, under the prominence of the cheekbone.

To sense the extent of the zygoma, cover the angular cheekbones with bunched fingers on each side. Move your index finger over the arch; place the middle finger on the outer corner of the eye socket, as the zygoma curves upward to join the frontal bone; and rest the ring and little fingers below the lower orbit of the eye and the thumb under the curve of the cheek. Your fingers encompass the zygomatic bone. Center your energy and notice any rhythmic movement of the zygoma. It is a complex result of movements of the frontal, maxilla, sphenoid, and temporal bones.

Now again become aware of the size and shape of the maxilla. Palpate from the inner orbit of the eye down both directly and diagonally to the entire gum line. The maxilla underlies the flesh here, bridging between the gums to form the arched roof of the mouth.

Nasal Bones

Bring three fingers to the bridge of your nose, so that the middle finger presses against the frontal bone and the other two fingers rest on each side of center. The nasal bones are just under these two fingers, giving shape to the bridge, joining the frontal and serving as attachment for the cartilage of the lower part of the nose.

Personal Areas

The face and the mouth are highly sensitive and intimately personal areas. Both pain and pleasure are felt intensely here. What is experienced and expressed around the mouth and face is felt to have a more direct connection to the heart and soul of the individual. As with the pelvis, physical trauma is likely to be bound up with emotional experience. It is important to work with special sensitivity, compassion, and patience around the mouth and face.

Initial Client Palpation

Usually, I recommend that this work be performed as part of a full treatment session. Even in a brief practice session, it is advisable to introduce and orient yourself through some more general body contact. For instance, touch the feet, shoulders, and head as in the listening stations. Give the client time to adjust to your presence and personal manner.

When I reach this place in my practice, I have worked with the releases of the body and the head. Then, with the client's permission, I ask her to shift on the table so that she is lying diagonally. Her head and shoulders move closer to the side where I will stand. For most procedures, I use

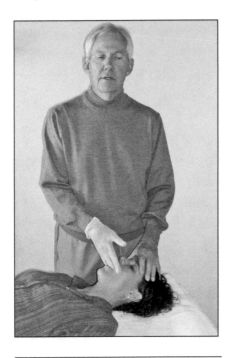

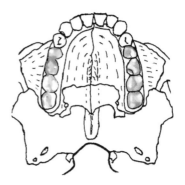

Figure 74a. Standing Position for Assessing the Maxillas and the Vomer.

Figure 74b. Contact Region on the Molars.

The wisdom tooth at each end may not be present.

either hand interchangeably. However, for work in the mouth, I usually use my dominant hand. I put an examination glove on that hand and stand parallel to the table, so that my shoulder and arm are at the level of her mouth. I lightly touch her frontal bone with the other hand, and let the gloved hand descend to her mouth.

With one hand on the frontal bone, gently place two fingers on the biting surfaces of her upper teeth, and encourage your client to relax her lower jaw. Though index and middle finger often feel more convenient to the therapist, the middle and ring fingers have the advantage of being closer to the same length. The palmar (inner) side of the fingers is used. The touch is soft.

Having made contact inside the mouth, I look to my own body posture. I want to stand erect and at ease. My neck, shoulders, and arms are relaxed. Energetically, I wish to be centered and grounded. There is seldom a need to look into the client's mouth as we work. The freer the body is, the freer and more sensitive the hand will be as we palpate and respond to sensations on the molars or the hard palate.

Stand for a few minutes, discovering how to be comfortable and relaxed in this position, and observing whatever is happening at the contact of fingers and teeth. Then, remove your hand and discuss how each of you felt. Considering this feedback, adjust your position again, place one hand on her forehead, and gently bring one finger to the roof of her mouth. Observe your own body posture and ease as well as the sensations emanating from this contact. In particular, let your hand, your arm, and even your vision relax. After a brief time, bring your hand away and discuss the experience with your client. Practice in this way a few times before going on to the release sections that follow.

The Maxillas

The maxillas are a key structure among the bones of the face and mouth because of their size and because of the many bones with which they articulate. In practice, we often find irregularity and constriction around the face and in the motion of the maxillas. At minimum, this is uncomfortable. Yet, constriction of sutures and joints may cause jaw, facial, or dental pain that has no apparent cause. Our goal is to aid the body in recovering its natural resilience in this area, restoring comfort and ease of movement.

We use a light touch. Remember that we are working with the natural healing capacity of the body. As pressure becomes too great, it stimulates the body's natural protective response. The tissue contracts and resists the therapist. The gentler and softer we are in presence and touch, the more we will feel. Likewise, the body responds more profoundly to a supportive touch.

Each of the four dysfunctions or displacements described here—flexion or extension; torsion; shear; and impaction—provides a means of assessing and releasing this region.

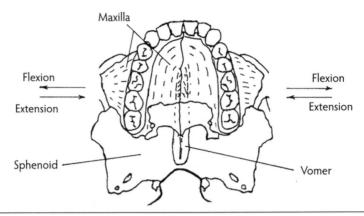

Figure 75. Flexion and Extension of the Maxillas. The motion of the craniosacral rhythm is transmitted from sphenoid through vomer to the upper surface of the roof of the mouth. Flexion: pressing downward, the vomer causes the maxillas to spread outward, as palpated on the molars. Extension: moving upward, the vomer draws the roof of the mouth with it, causing the molars to move inward.

Flexion or Extension Dysfunction

The fundamental approach is to observe the quality and range of the cranial rhythm. When we palpate maxilla movement on the molars, they move more into flexion (outward) or more into extension (inward) with each cycle. This is usually more pronounced on one side of the mouth.

Assessment

Stand next to the client with one hand contacting the upper molars as during the initial client palpation described above. The other hand is lightly placed on the client's forehead. Theoretically, this hand should monitor the craniosacral rhythm at the greater wings of the sphenoid. However, that position is often impractical and uncomfortable for client and therapist alike. The hand on the frontal bone serves to assess motion. It reassures the client and reduces the intensity of the contact within the mouth.

The rhythm within the cranial vault is communicated from the sphenoid to the upper jaw through the vomer. With each flexion of the rhythm, the sphenoid presses downward on the vomer, causing the molars to spread outward. At extension, with absorption of cerebrospinal fluid, the sphenoid and vomer return upward and the molars return inward. A component of the downward and upward motion of the sphenoid can be palpated, with light touch, on the frontal bone.

Monitor this cycle on the sphenoid or frontal bone and on the molars. Is the movement synchronized, the molars moving outward with flexion, inward with extension? Are flexion and extension equal in distance and strength? Any dysfunction is named for the direction of ease: is there a greater apparent travel in the direction of flexion or the direction of extension? Often this light touch is enough to bring release and balance. In practice, assess the vomer and then allow a pause before returning to the release procedure.

Releasing Procedure

With your fingers on the molars, follow the motions of flexion-extension. With your intention more than your fingers, emphasize movement in the direction of ease. Notice any sign of release. Then, after several cycles, emphasize motion in the restricted direction. Retain your light contact with the frontal bone during this entire procedure.

Lighten your touch; let the craniosacral rhythm resume and reevaluate. If sphenoid and maxillas are not synchronized in their movements, follow with your hand and finger positions, using light pressure on the molars to encourage synchronization: molars outward with flexion, inward with extension.

Torsion Displacement

Torsion is a twisting of the maxillas to one side, with the front of the bone moving the greater distance, seeming to hinge at the back of the palate. This may have its origin in an injury. However, when the condition is chronic, there may be no memory of a specific injury. Furthermore, facial constriction as an expression of life stress has the power to mimic or to recall a torsion pattern.

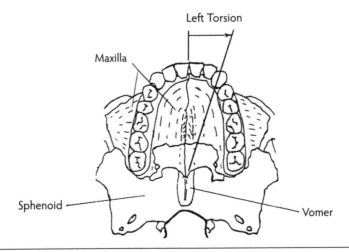

Figure 76. Torsion. The maxillas have been twisted to one side, usually due to a facial injury. The torsion may be to the right or to the left.

Assessment

Contact the forehead and upper molars as described for the initial client palpation. Body awareness and the comfort of both parties remains an important aspect of our client contact. You will have observed the cranial rhythm as expressed through the molars and on the frontal bone. If the rhythm is even, full, and in harmony, then there is probably no need to test for further dysfunctions. However, if some raggedness or lack of harmony remains, proceed with this assessment. It is also important for the beginning therapist to have the experience of testing lightly for this dysfunction.

With fingers in place, visualize and apply a subtle motion to one side in the horizontal plane, suggesting that the upper biting surface can twist in that direction. Allow several seconds for the bones to respond to this nonphysiological movement, then relax your hands and your touch.

Next, visualize and apply a twisting or torsion motion in the other direction. Any difference in the ease or degree of movement indicates a right or left torsion of the maxillas.

Start your torsion movement at the same point of the rhythmic cycle for each direction during assessment and release. That is, start each movement from the neutral (quiet) point after flexion or the neutral point after extension. Apply your touch gradually, remaining light enough that you do not stimulate resistance and contraction. The body responds more readily to a hint than to force.

Releasing Procedure

With one hand stabilizing on the frontal bone, visualize a torsion motion in the direction of ease, that is, in the direction of the apparent greater torsion. Assist this motion lightly with fingers on the molars and hold. Hold only a few seconds, or until you sense a release; then relax. Next, move into the direction of restriction. Pause briefly. Allow the craniosacral rhythm to resume for a few minutes before you reevaluate. Look for ease or a feeling of greater harmony rather than for exact balance.

Shear Displacement

Shear is a shifting of the entire structure of the maxillas to one side. It is as if the two bones could slide sideways, across the front of the face. Again, this may be due to an injury, or it may be part of a broader pattern of constriction and stress.

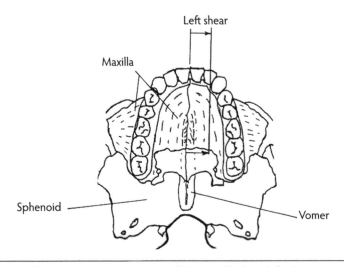

Figure 77. Shear. The entire structure of the maxillas has shifted to one side. The shear may be to the left or to the right.

Assessment

With the fingers of one hand on the upper molars and your other hand lightly resting on the frontal bone, visualize and move your hand and fingers directly to one side, with equal touch on the front and back of the teeth. Give time for a response. Relax, pause, and then move to the other side. If the movement response was greater in one direction than the other, then a right or left transverse shear of the maxillas is indicated. The touch and even the intent are very light.

Releasing Procedure

With hands in place as before, visualize and move in the direction of ease. Hold lightly but firmly until you sense a release. Relax, then move in the direction of restriction and through the restriction. The touch is light in each phase; it is as much a hint as it is an urging. Reevaluate after a few cycles of the craniosacral rhythm.

Impaction Displacement

At times, the maxilla bones seem jammed back against the palatines, the vomer, and the pterygoid processes of the sphenoid. There is a general quality of restriction in the region. It influences the cranial rhythm and may restrict nerve and fluid flow.

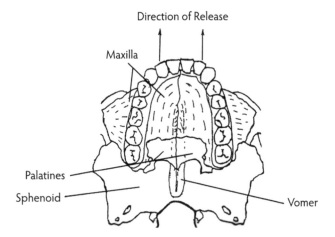

Direction of Release

Maxilla

Palatines

Sphenoid

Vomer

Figure 78. Impaction of the Maxillas. The maxillas have become lodged against the palatines, the vomer, and the sphenoid. Following the maxillas directly to the front performs both assessment and release.

Assessment

The maxillas are drawn forward. This may be done through friction against the upper molars by the two fingers that were used in the previous assessments. Or, the maxillas may be grasped through the gums above the front teeth. Use the thumb on the outer surface and one finger on the inside.

First, visualize the movement, and then gently draw the maxillas directly forward. Allow a few seconds for the bone structure to respond to this unusual motion. If the maxillas move easily forward, impaction is not a problem. If they do not, impaction may be present.

Releasing Procedure

If further release seems warranted, first pause and ensure that your client is comfortable continuing. Then renew your contact at the frontal bone and the molars or the maxilla. Rather than focus on the apparent restriction, look to your own posture. Ensure that your hands, arms, shoulders, and neck are at ease. Lighten your touch; remain centered and open. If the structure remains constricted, you may choose to apply a very light, steady forward motion. As the maxillas begin to respond, follow outward. Yet, remain very soft in your intent and touch. It is presence and support that encourages release. If constriction remains, then accept it for the moment and move on.

The Vomer

The vomer is a thin plate of bone that forms part of the nasal septum. In front of it, cartilage joins to complete the septum. Its long upper edge also joins the perpendicular plate of the ethmoid in completing the division of the nasal passage. The posterior end joins the body of the sphenoid. The rostrum, a projecting ridge on the sphenoid, fits into a cuplike depression on that upper end of the vomer. This provides security for the joint and flexibility of motion.

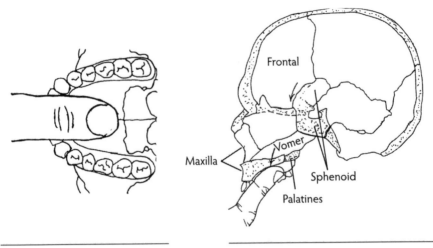

**Figure 79a. Finger Position
on the Vomer.**

Figure 79b. Side View.

The finger is positioned on the midline ridge at the roof of the mouth, at the suture of the maxillas, clear of the palatine bones. Arrows indicate the motion of flexion, the filling phase of the craniosacral rhythm. Extension is in the opposite direction.

At the floor of the nasal passage, the lower edge of the vomer rests on the roof of the mouth. It joins the maxillas and the palatine bones at their midline sutures. The vomer is thick enough to transmit the motions of the cranial vault to this extended midline of the hard palate. Yet it is thin enough to twist or buckle if extreme force is applied. Thus, the vomer may store the impact of a blow to the face, becoming impacted against the sphenoid or against the roof of the mouth.

If any restriction has been found in the motion of the maxillas, then it is important to also assess and release the vomer. If torsion or shear has been found in the maxillas, then the displacement of the vomer will often be in the same direction.

Client Palpation

Usually the client is lying face up on the treatment table; you can bring her head closer to you by having her lie diagonally on the table. Rest one hand lightly on the forehead. Use an examination glove or finger covering on the other hand for both of your protection.

Place the soft pad of one finger on the roof of the client's mouth, at its center along the midline ridge. The position is between the molars, toward but not as far back as the last molar. That is, your finger is on the suture between the maxillas, not quite as far back as the palatines.

As the body of the sphenoid presses downward with each flexion of the craniosacral rhythm, it transmits a rocking movement to the long plate of the vomer. The posterior section of the vomer presses downward on the suture between maxillas at the back of the mouth. With extension, the vomer and the roof of the mouth return upward. This motion may be felt by the finger: down and up.

The touch used in palpating and releasing the vomer is light and gentle, similar to that used in palpation of the sphenoid and less than that sometimes used in releasing the maxillas. Patience, presence, and sensitivity to the movements of the bones are as important as any physical pressure.

The motion of the cranial vault is monitored with the other hand on the frontal bone.

Flexion or Extension Dysfunction

Monitoring the motion of the vomer, discover if the cycle is equal on each side, or if it is longer ("easier") into flexion or extension. Focus your attention on the posterior portion of the suture between the maxillas to feel a down-and-up motion.

To release any dysfunction in the cycle, merely remain in contact with the vomer, gently urging it into an even cycle. When you feel the cycle is balanced, notice whether it is synchronized with the sphenoid or the frontal bone. Bring these motions together by a light suggestion with your finger and with your intention: downward together on flexion, upward together on extension.

Torsion Displacement

Torsion describes the situation when the vomer is twisted at its joint with the maxillas.

Let your finger rest along the midline suture as before, but a little further forward. Lightly monitor the craniosacral rhythm. At the neutral

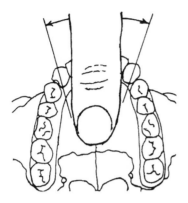

Figure 80a. Torsion Displacement of the Vomer. The finger tests for direction of ease and restriction with a twisting motion in each direction.

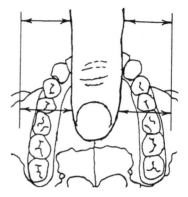

Figure 80b. Shear Displacement of the Vomer. The finger tests for direction of ease and restriction by lateral movement in each direction.

point after either flexion or extension, exert a light twisting motion with the finger on the roof of the mouth. You are transmitting torsion to the anterior base of the vomer. Gently stabilize the frontal bone as you do this and give enough time for the vomer to respond. It usually responds quite easily. If you do not notice a response, lighten the touch and try again.

Relax, allow the tissue to return to normal, and then exert a similar torsion in the other direction. If the response on one side is easier or greater, a torsion displacement in that direction is indicated.

Often, the assessing movement is enough to release the restriction. Be alert for signs of increased ease and fullness in the rhythm. If necessary, release further by gently moving and holding in the direction of ease until you sense a release. Then move in the other direction, gently drawing the vomer through the restriction.

Shear Displacement

Shear is the description used when the vomer appears to be displaced to one side or the other along its joint with the maxillas.

Lightly monitor the craniosacral rhythm. At the neutral point of either flexion or extension, visualize and exert a sideways motion with the finger on the roof of the mouth, transmitting a shear to the base of the vomer. Softly stabilize the frontal bone as you do this and give enough time for the vomer to respond.

Allow the tissue to return to normal, then apply a similar lateral motion in the opposite direction. If the response on one side is greater, then there is a shear displacement in that direction.

As with torsion, the assessment often provides the release. If not, then release this displacement by gently moving and holding in the direction of ease until you sense a release. Then move in the other direction, gently moving with the vomer through the restriction.

Impaction Displacement

The vomer is compressed against the sphenoid and its rostrum. It may also be wedged against the roof of the mouth.

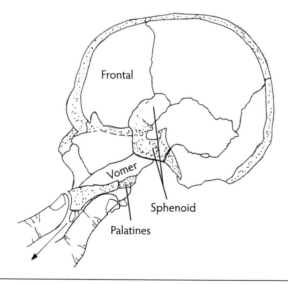

Figure 81. Impaction Relief. The finger at the roof of the mouth is aided by the thumb on the gums in front. The arrow between the fingers shows the direction of release, forward and down.

The connection between maxillas, vomer, and sphenoid feels rigid and inflexible. There is a lack of natural resilience in the tissues.

Lightly grasp the maxillas with one finger on the hard palate at its midline and the thumb on the outer lip. Restore space in this region by drawing the maxillas forward and down in one motion. Maintain gentle contact until you sense expansion and release. If you find no response, try one more time with a lighter touch and more relaxed inner energy.

This release may be used alone with clients who are very uncomfortable with work inside the mouth.

The Palatine Bones

The two palatine bones form the posterior portion of the hard palate, behind the maxillas. They are medial to the last molars on each side. If these wisdom teeth are missing, then the palatines are toward the center from the very back of the gums where these last molars would be.

Each bone is formed into a horizontal and a perpendicular plate. The horizontal plates join to present a small surface at the back of the hard

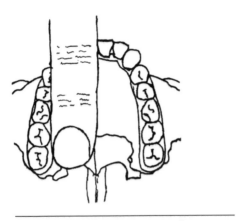

Figure 82a. Finger Position on the Palatine.

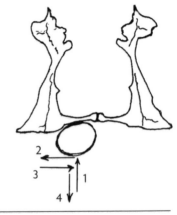

Figure 82b. Direction of Release.

Each side is released separately. Very light touch is used. The drawing on the right is a simplified view of the palatine bones from behind. The arrows indicate the directions followed in releasing the palatine. (See also figure 72a.)

palate. The perpendicular plates rise upward, fitting between the maxilla and the pterygoid processes of the sphenoid on each side. They make a small contribution to the orbit of each eye.

Very light touch is used in releasing the palatine bones. Make contact, then visualize motion in the required direction and follow. The intent is to restore resilience to each palatine bone at its sutures with the maxillas, the pterygoid processes, and the other palatine.

With one finger, follow the inside of the gums and molars to the last molar, or to the space on the gums reserved for that last molar. Slide the finger directly inward to the hard palate on that side.

You are in contact with the palatine bone through the soft tissue. Allow your hand, arms, and shoulders to relax. For the first moments merely observe whatever manifests itself through this contact. Then, step-by-step, visualize the idealized motions of release. With the lightest touch you can imagine, intend that the bone move in a superior direction. Whatever the response, visualize and follow the bone to the outside.

On sensing a response, return with the bone toward center, then below, to its starting point. You have followed the idealized pattern of palatine release at each of its sutures.

Use the same procedure to find and release the palatine on the other side of the midline. The palatine structure and sutures are very delicate, so it is better to work through visualization rather than effort.

The Zygomatic Bones

The zygomas, or cheekbones, give a unique shape to each person's face. Each zygoma joins the frontal bone near the end of the eyebrow and contributes to the outer or lateral orbit of the eye. Reaching back within the orbit, it connects with the greater wing of the sphenoid. This joint is covered by the layer of muscle at the temple. More obvious is its connection with the temporal bone. A narrow extension or process of the zygoma reaches back toward the ear to form the zygomatic arch with the temporal bone. The relatively small suture between temporal and zygoma can often be felt as a groove crossing the arch.

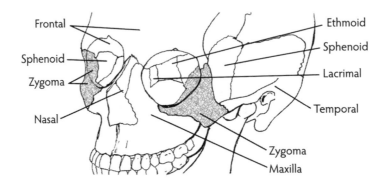

Figure 83. The Zygomatic Bones, the Ethmoid, and the Orbit of the Eye.
The zygomas determine the shape of the cheeks. This drawing shows the zygoma
as it articulates with the frontal, sphenoid, maxilla, and temporal bones in and around
the orbit of the eye. Note how the bone flares outward above the last molar.
The ethmoid contributes to the inner orbit and to the nasal passages.

The zygoma is firmly based on the maxilla, in a large suture which
extends downward and outward from the eye. It is the swelling outward of
the zygoma near this joint that lends a special shape to the face. Its joint
with the maxilla can often be felt as a small notch in the bone under the
eye. The surface of this joint is relatively large for the size of the bone.

Because of their prominence, the zygomas are vulnerable to injury.
When the tissues across the face are contracted, the zygomas may play a
role in limiting release in this region.

Palpation

Because they are connected to the maxillas as well as three cranial bones,
the motion of the zygomatic bones is complex. During flexion, or filling
of the cranial vault, the zygomatic bones may appear to widen in response
to the widening of the maxilla at the molars. During flexion, the zygomatic bones also appear to move downward with the greater wings of the
sphenoid and the frontal bone. These motions would be reversed as the
cranial vault shrinks during extension.

In practice, I do not attempt to differentiate these components. Sitting at the head of the table, I rest my forearms on the table surface. Then I bring my fingers to each side of the client's head so that my index finger touches the zygoma at the corner of the eye. My other fingers rest on the zygomatic arch and the jaw.

Assessment

Centering and grounding myself, I observe the quality of tissue and motion that are communicated through this touch. If I sense hardness or rigidity, I attempt to assist in the release of the zygomas and the tissues around them.

Release

The zygomas may be released from outside or from inside the mouth. To release from outside the mouth, I merely remain where I am, softly touching the zygoma at each side of the head. Often, this is sufficient to bring release and a sense of spreading.

When the constriction appears stronger, we can work as follows. Place one finger inside the mouth between the cheek and the gums at the last molar. Feel the flaring out of the bone above the finger. Place two or three fingers of your other hand on the zygoma from the outside. See that you are comfortable, with relaxed hands and arms.

With light touch, gently coax the zygoma outward in a diagonal direction. That is, the direction of release is combined lateral and anterior. Gently remain present until you sense an easing and releasing. Repeat the release on the other side.

Lightly contact the zygomas again from the outside. Note any change in the quality of their feel. Remaining present for a few moments may help the bones to find a new balance after the releases. If there is still some constriction or imbalance in this region, accept it for this session. A more complete release may occur some hours later, as the entire body integrates the effects of the session.

The Teeth

The teeth are discussed here because their release also requires a finger or hand covering, as in the previous releases. Usually, no such protection is necessary for the nasal bones.

Run a gloved finger slowly over the client's teeth. Notice any perception of energy focus, or of emptiness. Choose one or two teeth that seem to draw you most strongly.

Chose one tooth at a time. Gently hold the tooth between two fingers. Establish contact and awareness. Notice any change of energy, or an appearance of unwinding. Move with the tooth in your intention, but do not press the tooth in one direction or another. It is enough to remain present with your awareness and your energy. When the sense of motion or unwinding becomes quiet, the release is complete. Move to another tooth, if it seems appropriate. Discover how your client has felt during this experience. At times, another part of the body will experience release with the teeth.

The Nasal Bones

The nasal bones articulate with one another and with the perpendicular plate of the ethmoid bone at their midline suture. Nasal cartilage extends downward and forward from their ends to form the structure of the nose. The nasal bones join the frontal bone at their upper ends and the maxillas on each side. Our chief concern is that they are free in their articulations with the frontal bone and the ethmoid.

Sitting or standing to one side of the client's head, lightly contact the frontal bone with one hand. Place your thumb and index finger at the bridge of the nose, making contact with the two nasal bones beneath your fingertips. The traditional procedure recommends that you gently draw the nasal bones downward and outward, away from the frontal bone.

Often, it is enough to make gentle contact and remain there for a few minutes. Look for freedom of movement or a feeling of floating after the bones have a chance to respond to your presence.

If there is no apparent movement, lighten the touch; relax your arm, your fingers, and your intent. Observe any response. One side may be more tightly compacted than the other. These bones usually release easily. The position for the ethmoid and inner orbit may also ease the nasal bones.

The Ethmoid Bone and the Inner Orbit of the Eye

We often experience a general constriction around the eyes and face. This may be so mild that we are unaware of it. Yet, this constriction shows itself around and between the eyes during the release of the frontal bone. The following position helps soft tissue and joints to relax at the juncture of the many bones in that area. It touches and aids in the release of the maxilla, nasal, ethmoid, lacrimal, and frontal bones.

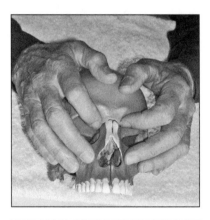

Figure 84a. Skeletal View of Ethmoid Contact.

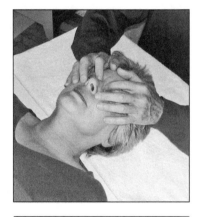

Figure 84b. Finger Positions on the Face.

In this position, the elbows rest on the table, while only the fingers touch the head and face.

Take a sitting position at the head of the table. Find support on the table for your elbows, and then rest your thumbs lightly on the frontal bone. Make sure that your arms and shoulders are comfortable and relaxed. Let the fingers of your hands rest on the client's cheeks on each side of the nose. Take a few moments in this position to let your arms, shoulders, and hands relax. The first few times, you may want to ask your client how this is for her. This is an external position from which we can sense the motion of the frontal and the maxillas.

After a few moments, bring your index fingers to the inner corner of each eye. Let the fingers gently touch close along the bridge of the nose, contacting the corner of the eye and the frontal bone. Merely remain relaxed and in position with a light touch at each point of contact. This is the release position. Softly remaining in place usually brings relief and comfort throughout the area.

Working Outside the Mouth

We can perform some of the above work outside the mouth, or with minimal intrusion. This is important for people who have difficulty tolerating any work inside the mouth.

The impaction release of the maxillas and the vomer relieves most dysfunctions with minimal intrusion into the mouth. Merely grasp the maxillas with thumb and fingers as is done for impaction of the vomer. From this position follow the procedures for release of the maxillas (directly forward), then the vomer (forward and downward on a diagonal).

Zygomas and maxillas can be palpated outside on the face, as described in the last sections above.

Rebalancing

After so much attention to the movement of the bones of the mouth and face, it is important to "back out" of the workspace. The ethmoid and inner orbit position described above helps bring a sense of wholeness and ease to this region. Usually, I also touch the sphenoid, not to adjust, but to bring a sense of support and completion. Then, I again make contact with the body and legs from a standing position. This helps the body to balance its energy and integrate changes. The first movements of the client after the session also help the body to integrate the many releases that have taken place.

Chapter 10

Integrating and Using Craniosacral Therapy

The intent of part 2 has been both to broaden and to deepen skills. The approach to general assessment and the specialized techniques for the cranial base, mouth, and face add to the skills that we may use in a session.

The material presented in chapter 5, "The Art of Touch," formalizes much that is embedded in the general tone of this book. I hope that this book will aid practitioners in developing an ever-deeper appreciation of the process that takes place between therapist and client.

I would like to conclude with a few more comments about the practice of therapy in general, and some thoughts on proceeding in a session.

The Learning Process

The hand positions and explanations presented in both parts make up the framework for learning craniosacral therapy. The qualities of presence, centeredness, and broad awareness imbue the work with a special spirit. Studying and practicing the release procedures forms a base for growing as a therapist. It is important to practice full sessions just as presented in these pages. Through each contact, we learn more than is written in a book. The therapist develops a deeper grasp of the power of each step through touch, through the hands, through experience. The knowledge and experience gained forms an ever-broadening foundation.

The inner qualities of awareness, presence, and respect carry the student beyond the formal structure of craniosacral therapy. With this approach, we learn to acknowledge as meaningful anything that the body manifests. Thus, we develop a special form of touch and communication. Touch becomes the guide to our interaction with the client. This quality of touch and presence goes beyond the name associated with this or that modality.

Despite all we learn from the form and the spirit of craniosacral, there is always more. The study of anatomy and physiology illuminates my understanding of what I am touching, what is occurring as the body releases. Other forms of gentle therapy and movement broaden my perspective on the body, the person, and the process.

Keep Open to Keep Learning

As we gain experience, we develop a base of knowledge and a set of expectations. The beneficial results of our work produce a feeling of confidence and competence. Praise from clients encourages our progress.

Yet, if I am too certain of my knowledge, it can interfere with continued progress. If I think I know exactly what will occur, then I am in awe of my own knowledge, but cut off from experiential reality. The knowledge, the experience, the results, and the thanks contribute to a foundation. Throughout life, we are building on that base. Openness to new possibilities, to new patterns and relationships ensures that I am actually with the new client. My knowledge and experience are available in the background; they offer valuable guidance, but not every answer in every situation. The answer reveals itself in the process that occurs at this moment with this person.

In each encounter, I acknowledge the importance of moving from emptiness and openness rather than from fixed theory or experience alone.

What I Look for During a Session

In the first years of my work with craniosacral, I began the session with arcing (described in chapter 6). It enabled me to observe areas of focus and freedom along the client's body. When I looked again after the session, I saw not focus, but flow up and down the body, balance from side to side, and a quality of calm. Eventually, these qualities became my goals. The symptoms, the areas of tissue hardness and constriction, became less interesting than the return of muscle softness, resumed flow through regions of the body, and a feeling of quiet and inner harmony. Thus, I am working with a broad view, looking beyond symptoms, not so perturbed by evidence of stress and trauma. I have experienced repeatedly that the body can recover balance, regain flow, and recover flexibility. I support and encourage rather than lead.

I look for many small releases over the whole body rather than a major breakthrough in one location. Small changes are easier to integrate than major changes. Once the body begins to change, the process of integration and adaptation continues long after a session.

Before concluding a session, I may check back to places I haven't touched, or that did not release fully at first. If some constriction remains, I accept it. There may be an important sequence or timing for letting go that I do not yet recognize.

When nothing is happening, when a place is not moving, I lighten my touch and give more space. When I feel stuck and unclear, I also lighten and give space. Or I move. Often, beginning to move my hand or getting up and moving a step helps me to gain a broader perspective, to "see" what to do next.

The Significance of Patterns

No chronic misalignment or constriction is simple and isolated. The body compensates for a restriction of function in one area by adapting neighboring joints and tissue. A new pattern of movement and flow develops. As time goes by, this pattern extends further. Craniosacral therapy works well with chronic patterns because it operates broadly. By touching all of the diaphragms, we reach the whole body. By offering space and support, we encourage the body to open connections that we neither see nor feel.

Touch and hold the quiet or "empty" places. Touch and support can bring life and flow, renewing integration with the whole body. Wait for motion, flexibility, a sense of widening or softening. A part that had relaxed may contract as you move to a new location. Accept this and wait for a new balance and release to occur from a distance.

Words and Intention

Words and even thoughts are powerful tools in the therapy session. Often when an area is very still and slow to soften, the tissue responds to a few words. For instance, at times the neck muscles are tight, making the atlanto-occipital release slow and painful to both therapist and client. I may quietly explain what I am doing. I speak in an objective manner, descriptive rather than judgmental.

For example, "I am holding my fingers this way to help the muscles release. As they soften, the vertebrae can gain more space between them."

Or I may more directly acknowledge the role of the body, saying, "These muscles have been working hard to help you. They can rest for a while, and become firm anytime there is need."

Or, "There is no need to relax any more than is safe."

Often a release takes place with or soon after such words. Yet, such words cannot be used as a mere formula. I must have enough respect for the inner process of the client to actually mean what I say.

In working with the bones of the head, mouth, or face, it is often helpful to lead with your intention. That is, make contact with your hands, center yourself, and observe the movement of the structures you are holding. Then form a clear intention of the release process before beginning. You may find that the bones lead you through the release. If you have difficulty partway through the release, maintain contact, but center your energy and lighten your touch. You may again visualize the smooth, balanced motion that appears after a release, but accept the pathway that the body chooses to reach that state.

Whether this relaxed acceptance helps the therapist, or communicates with the client on a nonconscious level, it is often beneficial. Perhaps the hands work more knowingly. However, experience shows that the constricted tissue of the client is sensitive to the intent and the openness of the therapist.

The Sacrum, the Pelvis, and the Back

Many of us experience pain somewhere in the back. The symptom may be anywhere from the pelvis to the head. When I palpate along the back, usually I find the muscles are tight all along from lower back to neck and occiput. Each of us has a place where the constriction finds a voice. Where it really starts is not so clear. The entire back is involved, no matter where the pain is felt. So, we work all along the back.

At times the sacrum and pelvis feel very hard and heavy, so that it is painful to remain directly in contact for any length of time. Be careful of yourself. You can work around the area. Work on the pelvis from the side, above, and below. Include the shoulders and head.

Taking Care of the Therapist

The health and well-being of the therapist are as important as that of the client. As I learn to care for others, I also learn to care for myself. The therapeutic process, like life, is a process of mutual learning, of mutual healing. Within this process, I learn my capabilities, my strengths, and my weaknesses. I discover more clearly my humanity and learn to honor this process in myself as I am learning to be guided by it in my clients.

In learning my capabilities, I discover what I can handle. I learn to say no when it is important for my well-being and to rest rather than do sessions when my energy is depleted.

Within a session, I repeatedly reestablish my awareness of my own energy, flow, and vulnerabilities. When a strong emotion or sensation comes to me during the session, I ask myself, is this from the client or from me? In fact, my sensitivity and vulnerability prepare me to be responsive to the client. Many things that I feel in a session resonate with my issues. Yet, the client may experience them differently than I do. The resolution for the client will be unique to that person. My experience helps me to be sensitive, but I want to remain open enough that I do not impose my problems or their solution on my client.

In my private life, I seek to consult my body. What is right for me? What attracts, what repels, what energizes, what depletes? I attempt to learn to live so that I honor what my total self is telling me. As I feel this working in my life, I gain confidence that it works for others, each in their own way.

I get sessions from others, craniosacral and other forms of therapy. As I nourish myself in this way, I also discover more fully what therapy is all about, how it feels, how it functions.

I learn how to ask for help and to receive help and support from others. I learn to recognize the part of myself that does not want to receive, to open, or to share. I extend respect and compassion for that part in myself, just as I offer it to others.

A Sacred Way

After years of experience, I am convinced that we perceive only a small fraction of what occurs as we touch. Yet, the work is very effective on many levels of the total person. Because I cannot see and rationally explain all that happens, there is a feeling of mystery and magic about the results. I have heard that in craniosacral therapy we contact special, sacred aspects of the person. From that viewpoint, craniosacral becomes a sacred science.

Craniosacral therapy has a very special place in my life. Yet, I believe that it is no more sacred than any other therapeutic modality. It is the therapeutic process itself that may be considered sacred; it is the mutually respectful client-therapist interaction that deserves awe and reverence. In the end, it is our involvement in the therapeutic process that is our greatest teacher. Our adherence is not to one modality or one school of thought, but to the process of healing. We are privileged to participate in that.

TREATMENT PROTOCOL

THE LISTENING STATIONS	Standing:	Ankles (front and back)
		Thighs
		Hips
		Ribs
	Sitting:	Shoulders
		Neck & Occiput
		Sphenoid
RELEASING THE BODY		Pelvic floor
		Lumbosacral joint
		Sacroiliac joints
		Respiratory diaphragm
		Upper thorax
		Hyoid region
		Atlanto-occipital joint
THE CRANIAL RELEASES		Mastoid process
		Frontal
		Parietal
		Sphenoid
		Temporal ear pull
		Temporal 3 finger
		Mandible
		Occiput—CV-4

Arnold, *Rhythm and Touch*

The above outline may be copied and used as a reminder during your early practice sessions.

Therapeutic Dialog in Craniosacral Therapy

As therapists, we provide a safe, supportive space for our client. Within this secure space, the client is free to sink into a relaxed, receptive state, similar to the alpha state of meditation or hypnosis. Now the sympathetic nervous system can reduce its labors; the parasympathetic system is free to resume the functions of nurturance, repair, and strengthening of the immune system. Thus the client's healing and reorganizing capability is reactivated. This inner capability makes possible the most profound sequences of therapeutic release. Healing occurs from within, directed by the natural resources of body and spirit.

In craniosacral, we assist this reawakening through special qualities of touch and presence. The touch is light, supporting the inner process. Presence and awareness go hand in hand. Presence means being here, now, in this place with this person. It also means being awake and aware toward self, conscious of my changing physical and emotional comfort.

A state of quiet and trust opens the channels of intuitive communication. Within this quiet I am more sensitive to the gentle messages passing body to body, spirit to spirit, heart to heart.

Craniosacral was born of a manipulative tradition, in which the therapist directed the healing. Since its inception, we have learned that gentle support is more powerful than pressure or direction. Muscles and tissues ease, joints recover resilience, the spirit is uplifted. The phases of recovery unfold from within. Experience has taught us how to participate effectively in this silent unfolding, attentive to the inner voices of both client and therapist.

Conversation in Therapy

Conversation is a natural part of the client-therapist interchange. Words can express inner experience. As companions to presence and touch, they can further stimulate inner flow and unfolding. Our challenge is to discover how to use dialog effectively in this exchange, how to use words harmoniously in concert with the inner unfolding.

An effective use of speech mirrors the quality of our physical touch and presence. Therapeutic dialog retains the light touch of the hands. We are in touch, without pressure: respectful of the client, trusting the unseen process, giving space, following and supporting.

Conversation is not sustained, but intermittent. Moments of silence nourish awareness; effective speech flows from awareness.

Introducing Verbal Communication

Craniosacral can be a very quiet experience. Many people enjoy sinking into a deep silence, remaining there for most of the session. This is a very nurturing experience in which the body, and all its potencies, accomplishes wonders of relaxation, energetic reorganization, and pain relief.

Yet, verbal feedback is important, even with a person whom we know well. It is even more important if the client is experiencing pain. Then, the reaction to touch can vary a lot at different places on the body.

Starting

At the beginning of a session, I usually ask: "What is it that you hope for from this session? What would you like to tell me about your body?"

Asking these questions may seem redundant with someone we know. Yet, each time, it gives that person the chance to think about and express what is happening now. It encourages the individual to formulate an intention. The intention may be large or small. It does not matter.

The question encourages the client to recognize that choice is possible. The therapist does not take the client's intention as an imperative for the session. Rather, it serves the client as an inner suggestion to the self of hopes and desires.

Feedback: Sharing the Experience

Verbal feedback is very important to us as therapists. It is impossible to know intuitively everything that the client feels and experiences. I may feel comfortable and tuned in, but the touch or closeness is stirring up a difficult sensation for the client. So I simply ask: "How is this for you?" Or, "What are you experiencing (feeling, noticing)?" The question is simple and open, inviting any comment from the person on the table.

Or I may ask specifically, "Is this hand position comfortable?"

The client wants feedback, too. Sometimes it is more effective to describe than to question. Here, the choice of words is important.

I might feel hardness, constriction, or pressure. I want to formulate these impressions so that what I say is informative yet constructive. I may say: "I notice some tightness in these muscles." This signals that the constriction is relative, not absolute.

I may rephrase the observation, using words that put the constriction in a broader context.

"This region has been working very hard to strengthen or protect you. Now it can take the opportunity to relax."

"It has been doing its job. Now it can take a little rest."

"This region can experiment with another level of holding."

Sometimes the therapist experiences a strong emotion or visual image. These may be stimulated by the client's inner process. Therefore, they may be a helpful indication of an unspoken theme. On the other hand, such experiences are colored by the therapist's own life experience and personality. Thus, I cannot always be certain that my impression is helpful exactly as I feel it. In a few words, I can briefly mention or wonder about a theme. Yet, I do it tentatively. I tone down the strength of my feeling, leaving it to my client to supply her own coloring and intensity. I do not try to build on my impression, but simply accept whatever the client says in response.

Descriptions and Hints

"This region can take the opportunity to relax, to take a break from its efforts."

"These muscles have been working very hard. Now they have a chance to recall how to relax."

"These muscles have been working for you. They are not an enemy; they just need help to recognize other possibilities, to recall a fuller range of activity."

This way of speaking contains a variety of suggestions. I acknowledge that the muscles have been working for the body. Tightness and holding is one of the functions of body tissue. The goal of constriction is to protect or strengthen. But when we have worked under repeated stress, muscles and tissue often fail to return to a fully relaxed condition. They retain a readiness to tighten, to protect.

Now, in the security of this session, the muscles can recover a fuller range: they are able to be both loose and tight.

I note the possibility, the opportunity of remembering a full range. Even when I am initially struck by hardness or constriction, I speak in a way that offers appreciation and opportunity.

Thus, description may be neutral or include hints. Often a simple objective description results in movement and opening. Fewer words are more powerful than many; "less is more."

Cue Words

When we use cue words, we simply repeat a single word or a short phrase from something the client has said.

When we use the client's own words, we support and empower the experience of the client. This usage stimulates rather than interrogates.

The client may describe a feeling or memory. A simple repetition of one word shows the interest and receptiveness of the therapist. One word may prompt a more detailed explanation. Simultaneously, it often ushers in a broader physical release.

The client says, "I have an image of my father when I was a child." I respond, "Your father" or "When you were a child."

The client says, "I am feeling lighter (more relaxed, at ease)." I may respond, "Yes." *Yes* accepts, affirms the client's experience, deepening it.

Or, I may merely respond, "Lighter." This may stimulate a fuller description of the client's experience.

Suggestions and Recommendations

Ordinary comments in social situations have a certain power. They act on both the conscious and the unconscious mind, especially if the recipient is in a vulnerable state. For example, a question may hide a suggestion. Do you feel tired? Do you feel good? Do you feel pain? Do you enjoy this? The embedded suggestions are: feel tired; feel good; feel pain; enjoy this.

This is why warnings and prohibitions have a paradoxical effect: they plant in the mind the exact thing which is not desired.

Within the deepened receptivity of therapy, the words of the therapist have an even more powerful suggestive effect. A description, a cue, or a hint becomes a suggestion when the conscious and unconscious mind takes it in and works with it. Simple words and phrases stay in the mind, influencing thought and feeling.

Thus, I want to use words that encourage and affirm. These words are based on what is there, what is happening. They help the client to recognize a firm foundation from which to move onward.

The client has mentioned, "I am beginning to feel that old pain in my shoulder." If I use the word *pain,* it can affirm the client's experience. But it may serve as a reminder and trigger for pain. So, when I feel some release has occurred, I merely say, "The shoulder?"

Many constructive suggestions are contained in the verbal descriptions, cues, and hints offered here. These words and phrases acknowledge what either of us may be experiencing. They encourage by affirming the efforts the body and mind have been making. They do not overwhelm and discourage by offering advice and personal viewpoints; they are minimal and recognize the significance of small change.

The Goal of Dialog

Words engage the rational mind. In our culture, we often disregard the evidence of our senses as we engage in thought and speech. As therapists we wish to remain harmonious with the body process as we dialog with the client.

Therapy does not happen overnight. Change is an organic process. It comes from within. As therapists, we enjoy finding out more of what the client thinks and feels. But the greater goal of our touch and dialog is to support the inner process of healing. This extends far beyond what I can perceive, understand, or describe. It is important to know and respect that I do not know all that is happening within the client.

The therapeutic process is active within each of us. Through my own healing process, I gain a deeper insight and trust in the possibility of healing for others. Awareness of myself and my process is the foundation for understanding the process in others. The process of healing is learned from inside, as I witness my life, and it is learned in relationship with each client, as I participate in that other healing process.

Furthermore, as I learn to apply these qualities in communicating with my client, I learn to speak more softly and effectively to myself, with encouragement and trust.

Conclusion

Here is a summary of the communication philosophy presented in this book. These points are useful for our type of therapy, whether we are using words or working in silence.

1. I recognize that the symptoms are the result of the natural capabilities of muscle, tissue, and spirit. The body is a friend, working for the person.

2. I express gratitude for these efforts.

3. I suggest that this is a moment when the tissue can experiment with relaxing as well as holding.

4. My suggestions are minimal. This relaxation is something for the moment; the tissue still retains the ability to be tight or resistant when it is useful.

5. My suggestions emphasize positive capability. They are small steps within the power of the organism.

6. I learn from my personal healing journey. That helps me to have compassion, patience, and trust, with myself and with others.

Glossary of Terms

altered state of consciousness. A mental state in which ordinary awareness and thought processes are modified. In an altered state, a person may become more or less aware of physical sensations or of body functions. The sense of time may greatly change. Pain may disappear or intensify. Awareness is usually more inward than outward.

anterior. Directed forward or situated toward the front of the body.

arcing. An assessment procedure described by John Upledger. The hand of the practitioner appears to be drawn to specific parts of the body, focal points of energy or restriction.

ASIS. Acronym for anterior superior iliac spine, the forward point of the hip bone on each side of the body.

bregma. A point at the top front of the skull where the coronal and sagittal sutures meet, where both parietal bones join the frontal bone.

caudal. Situated or directed toward the tail or lower part of the body.

cephalad. Toward the head.

coronal suture. The cranial suture where the anterior edges of the parietal bones join the posterior edge of the frontal bone. It extends upward from behind and above the temple area to bregma, at the sagittal suture.

CV-4. Compression of ventricle four. A technique for inducing a still point by means of gentle pressure on the occiput.

diaphragm. The muscular partition between the abdominal and thoracic cavities that functions in respiration. More generally, any membrane that divides or separates. Thus the term is also applied to other regions in the body where there may be a natural, structural restriction of communication and flow, such as at the pelvic floor and at the thoracic opening, the place where the neck meets the torso.

direction of energy. A treatment procedure related to the V-spread of William Sutherland. It is thought that the therapist's hands can direct energy through a symptomatic region in order to assist release.

directions of movement. Terms of position and motion that are always in relation to the body itself without reference to gravity, earth, or sky. For example, *down* means down the length of the body, toward the feet, even if the client is doing a headstand. *See also names of individual directions*

dural tube. The extension of the dura mater from the cranial vault into and down the spinal column. The protective lining for the spinal cord within the spinal column.

dura mater. Latin for "tough mother." The strong connective membrane providing part of the protective environment of the brain and spinal cord. It lines the cranial vault and forms a sleeve which extends down the spinal canal.

energy cyst. A term devised within a medical setting to describe the stagnation of fluid and energetic movement within a limited area of the body. It is usually associated with chronic restriction and pain.

extension. The straightening of the sphenoid and occiput from the sphenobasilar joint. Applied to changes throughout the head and body that are associated with absorption of cerebrospinal fluid and contraction of the cranial vault, the term can be confusing because it generally describes an inward motion. *See also* flexion; flexion and extension

falx cerebri. A fold of the dura mater that partially separates the two sides of the brain and attaches at the ethmoid and frontal bones, along the sagittal suture.

flexion. The bending downward of the sphenoid and occiput from the sphenobasilar joint. Applied to changes throughout the head and body that are associated with filling and expansion of the cranial vault, the term can be confusing because it is generally an outward motion. *See also* extension; flexion and extension

flexion and extension. The terms used by William Sutherland to describe the motion of the sphenoid in relation to the occiput. *See also* extension; flexion

foramen (*plural* foramina). An opening through or between bones for the passage of blood vessels or nerves.

foramen magnum. The large circular opening at the base of the skull, in the occipital bone, which allows the spinal cord and its protective membranes to enter the spinal column.

full protocol. *See* protocol

hypertonia, hypertonicity. A degree of tissue excitation and tension that is above the ordinary level necessary for functioning.

impaction. A displacement that occurs when bones are jammed against each other so that motion is severely restricted.

inferior. Situated below or directed downward, away from the top of the head, toward the feet.

lambda. The point at the back of the skull where the sagittal suture meets the lambdoid suture and both parietal bones join the occiput, just above the occipital prominence in the back of the skull.

lambdoid suture. The cranial suture where the posterior edges of the parietal bones join the upper edge of the occiput at the back of the skull. This joint extends downward and to the sides in a diagonal, forming the Greek letter lambda: Λ.

lateral. Situated to the side or directed outward from the middle toward the side.

listening stations. Locations along the legs and body where the craniosacral rhythm is noted at the beginning of a therapy session.

mastoid process. A rounded projection of the temporal bone behind the ear.

medial. Situated or directed toward the center, inward from the side toward the middle.

mid-sagittal. Used to describe a view in the front to back plane, exactly at the midline of the body part. *See also* sagittal

neutral zone. A period during the regular cycle of the craniosacral rhythm during which the sphenoid appears to be at rest, fully in flexion or in extension.

occiput. The occipital bone, forming the back of the head. It joins the spinal column.

palmar. The palm side of the hand.

palpate. To feel or sense with the hands.

periosteum. The membrane covering each bone, a type of connective tissue.

pia mater. Latin for soft or sweet mother. The fine protective membrane covering every surface of the brain and spinal cord.

posterior. Situated behind or directed backward, toward the back of the body.

protocol. The steps comprising a full session of craniosacral therapy at the introductory level, also called *full protocol, treatment protocol,* or *ten-step protocol.* The complete protocol includes the listening stations and the releases of the body and the cranium.

release. *See* therapeutic release

sagittal. Used to describe a plane dividing the body into right and left parts. *See also* mid-sagittal

sagittal suture. The joint between the parietal bones at the top of the head, extending from bregma on the coronal suture to lambda on the lambdoid suture.

shear. A sideways displacement of two objects along the surface where they meet.

solar plexus. The pit of the stomach. In this book *solar plexus* is used in this broad, informal sense.

sphenobasilar synchondrosis. The joint between the sphenoid and occiput, connected by a slightly flexible pad of cartilage.

squamous suture. The joint on each side of the head between the temporal bone, which hosts the ear, and the parietal bone, which is situated above and behind the temporal bone.

still point. The apparent temporary cessation of the craniosacral rhythm during craniosacral therapy. The use of this term has been extended to any period of deep quiet and relaxation during any therapy session.

superior. Situated above or directed upward, away from feet, toward the top of the head.

temple. The flat area on the side of the face, just behind the corner of the eye and above the zygomatic arch.

temporal bone. The bone on each lower side of the head which provides the ear canal and the joint with the jaw.

temporomandibular joint. The joint between the temporal bone and the mandible (lower jaw), just in front of the ear canal.

ten-step protocol. A term often used to refer to the steps of a full craniosacral therapy session. The term probably originated at a time when only ten steps were in use. *See also* protocol

tentorium cerebelli. A stabilizing fold of the dura mater extending across the cranial vault above the cerebellum. It attaches on each side at the petrous portion of the temporal bone and crosses the lower end of the falx cerebri.

therapeutic pulse. A pulsation beneath the therapist's hand or fingers that may feel like the cardiac pulse, but unlike the heart pulse rises, peaks, and dissipates.

therapeutic release. A process occurring within the body tissue that eases constriction and resumes the flow and interchange with nearby tissue and organs.

torsion. A twisting out of a usual position.

treatment protocol. *See* protocol

unwinding. The part of the release process when a body part, supported by the therapist, moves through a pattern of its own choice. Sometimes accompanied by memories, insights, or metaphorical images regarding the source of the dysfunction.

Vipassana meditation. A form of meditation in which the goal is calm acceptance of all inner experience. It is usually practiced by sitting quietly and "watching" the breathing, alternating with walking with the same quiet inner awareness.

zygoma (*plural* zygomas *or* zygomata). The cheekbone on each side of the face.

zygomatic arch. The prominent ridge extending forward on each side of the head, from the ear canal to the upper cheek.

INDEX

ABOUT THE AUTHOR

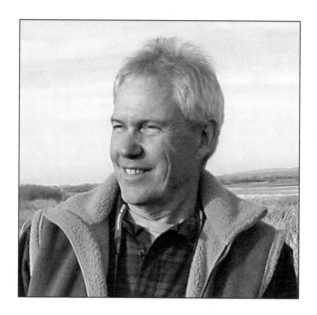

Anthony P. Arnold brings to his work almost forty years of experience and inquiry into the field of therapy. After doctoral studies at the University of Chicago, he worked for many years as a clinical psychologist. As his career evolved, he studied the issues of working with the unconscious in hypnosis and in ordinary life. Finally, he pursued his interest in the interaction of mind, body, and spirit through the study of Shiatsu, craniosacral therapy, and massage.

He lives and practices in Santa Fe, New Mexico. For more information, you may visit his Web site: www.rhythmandtouch.com.